# Keep My Son

A Mother's Unprecedented Battle and Victory Over
her Son's Mental Illness

Diane Borders

Original Cover Art Work by Cynthia Rutherford
Cover Design by Tyler Borders

ISBN-10: 0-9975397-2-0
ISBN-13: 978-0-9975397-2-1

# Dedication

———✦———

This book is dedicated to my amazing husband who is my soul mate, the love of my life, and my best buddy. I can't imagine doing life with anyone else. You always encourage me to go for what I believe in and stand behind me 110%. Thank you for being in my corner, cheering me on to retire and pursue writing this book. It meant a change in vocation. Not many husbands would be so open to such a major life change, but you optimistically launched me out of my comfort zone and into this new world.

Also, Daniel, Tyler, and Karis, each of you are precious and make my life rich beyond measure. Our family is only complete when we're all together. I cherish each of you with my whole being. Your contributions to the making of this book were immense. Your insight, direction, and artistic suggestions were immeasurable in its preparation. You will always have my heart.

You are all brave for letting me tell this story.

# Table of Contents

# Foreword

My grandfather was born in 1896. He grew up on a western ranch, riding horses and wagons for transportation. It wasn't until he was well into elementary school that he saw his first car. He married in 1919 and he and my grandmother left on a cargo ship for the shores of eastern India, a trip that took over a month, where he started a mission program including hospitals and clinics.

By the end of his career, he was the chief administrator of a group of some 400 mission hospitals and clinics around the world. He could rapidly travel via modern jet to almost any location on the globe in only a few hours. What a change! In one lifetime, the world of transportation was radically altered; Horses and buggies to cars and jet airplanes.

I imagine when he saw the first horseless buggy going down the dirt street in his small town, he had absolutely no idea of the dramatic changes that would be taking place in the world of transportation within just a relatively few years: Interstate freeways, huge modern airports, 747s and A380s.

Once the petroleum-based motor was invented, the future changes were already implicit within the concept. Yet few had the vision to see what was coming. Even twenty or thirty years later, it would have been challenging to see the future interstate highways and jet aircraft.

The next major revolution was computer and information technology. It developed slowly for many years, but reached a major push around 1990 with the development of the Internet. Information could now be obtained from distant locations instantly. What I used to have to travel to major university medical libraries to read, I could now get on my computer via the Internet. Information of all sorts became available to everyone. In the field of medicine, especially, information was no longer solely the domain of medical professionals.

PubMed was initiated in January of 1996. With PubMed, anyone can easily search through virtually all medical research data. One no longer has to travel to some medical library to find information as it is all available on one's own computer. At first, there was a limited amount of information available on PubMed. But today, most medical research is available on the site.

One other point here is that there is so much information coming out in research journals that no one in the world can begin to encompass or understand even a small amount of the research. And unfortunately, most doctors simply don't have the time to read the medical literature either at all or especially outside of their specific field of interest.

One of the amazing changes taking place quite rapidly in the field of medicine is its democratization. Since it is increasingly impossible for any physician to keep up with the wide amount of information coming out, non-medical people are taking it upon themselves to research issues that relate to them or their families. Some are doing an excellent job of understanding the issues they're facing and are truly finding better answers than their physicians are able to offer.

This in itself can create some friction.

Historically, doctors have been trained to see themselves as the ones who know. They have gone through long and rigorous training. No one else can know and understand what they do, or so they think. Therefore, many doctors find themselves going on the defensive when patients come to them asking questions that go beyond their understanding. It can become especially difficult when a "patient" comes in with suggestions for finding a better diagnosis in particularly difficult health issues, or when the doctor is told of some other mainstream or even integrative approaches to the patient's disease process.

What I hear all too often when talking with the people who come to consult with me is that doctors will completely shut them off when they begin to ask questions or make suggestions the doctor is unfamiliar with. Sometimes they will be subtly made fun of, or the doctor will just disconnect from them.

This should not happen.

A realistic, or should I say humble, doctor will not take any offense at all. S/he should recognize the Internet provides answers (or at least thoughts, questions, and ideas) to anyone who goes searching. Since no doctor can possibly know everything about any field, s/he should welcome interacting with a motivated patient who wants to work cooperatively.

As Emma Hill, Editor of The Lancet, one of the most prestigious medical journals in the world, wrote, "Every patient is an expert in their own chosen field, namely themselves and their own life." We could tag on "and health" and perhaps clarify the intent of her statement further.[i]

A wonderful book which explores some of these issues of doctor and patient relationships was written by an eminent cardiologist, Eric Topol, titled *The Patient Will See You Now*. Dr. Topol shows that some of these attitudes have been built into the education and training of doctors for centuries and millennia. The American Medical Association (AMA) used to be considered the society for all physicians. That has changed with time. Now, less than one quarter of American doctors belong.

But when the AMA was founded, its code of ethics included statements like the following.

"10. A patient should never weary his physician with a tedious detail of events or matters not appertaining to his disease.

11. The obedience of a patient to the prescriptions of his physician should be prompt and implicit. *He should never permit his own crude opinions as to their fitness, to influence his attention to them.* (my italics)

12. A patient should never send for a consulting physician without the express consent of his own medical attendant (meaning, a patient not satisfied with the care she is receiving for her knee pain, for instance, should not make an appointment to see an orthopedist for a second opinion without her primary doctor's consent).

17. The benefits accruing to the public and indirectly from the active and unwearied beneficence of the profession, are so numerous and important, that physicians are justly entitled to the utmost consideration and respect from the community."[ii]

The AMA had inculcated a sense of superiority in physicians making it sometimes difficult for them to see the wisdom and insight of their patients. This is increasingly true as we get into the field of genomics, which is in some ways the subject of this book

Very few doctors really understand genetics in any great depth. This is a new and rapidly developing field. For many, there is simply not the time to research and understand. Yet the possibilities in that field are momentous. Since doctors generally know very little about it, how might individuals facing disease themselves or in their families make use of the information now available to them?

First, one must have access to the information. This access has been opposed by groups like the AMA.

Dr. Topol has been working to improve access to information for people in general. In 2013, he had an interview with the WSJ regarding the access people have to their own genetic information. The AMA at the time was lobbying to obstruct that availability. Following is a quote from that interview:

*"WSJ: What are roadblocks for moving to this new world?*

DR. TOPOL: A core problem is the medical profession. The average time it takes for a significant innovation to become standard clinical practice is 17 years...

But what has really gotten me stirred up is the issue of whether patients should have access to their own health data. The AMA [American Medical Association] was lobbying the government that consumers should not have access directly to their DNA data, but that it has to be mediated through a doctor. The AMA did a survey of 10,000 doctors, and 90% said they have no comfort using genomics in their clinical practice. So how could they be the ultimate mediator by which the public gets access to their DNA data? That really speaks to medical paternalism.

The fact that consumers will have this ability to have themselves—their genome sequence, their lab tests, their tissues—digitized on their smartphones and their social networks will reboot the way doctors interact with patients." [iii]

Thankfully, it seems that access to this data is increasingly available to each of us.

We don't have time to explore the historical attitudes of doctors toward patients further. Organized medicine, as epitomized by the AMA, has tried to prevent individuals from having access to their own biological data. But most doctors have very little idea of what to do with easily available genetic information from sources such as

23andme. This is the context in which many intelligent, inquisitive, and diligent people find themselves.

Second, when we have access to this complicated genetic information, what do we do with it? How do we understand this information? It is here that we find the work of people like Diane Borders standing out like a bright star on a dark night.

I've known Diane for over 20 years and I find the work she is doing inspiring, enlightening, and brave. She is one who epitomizes the intelligent, inquisitive, and diligent researcher determined to find answers. In this case, her goal was to find answers for her son, whose story is told in these pages.

My hat is off to Diane for her hard work, her study, her learning how to work with the medical profession and, most importantly, figuring out how to get her son well. In spite of the roadblocks attempted by groups like the AMA, it is important to learn how to work with doctors to accomplish the best outcome. Diane has maintained an attitude of cooperation and mutual enlightenment with doctors willing to acknowledge that they don't know it all and who appreciate input from a non-medical colleague.

The kind of thinking outlined here may be the kind of thinking necessary for many with chronic health challenges, whether they be mild, moderate, or severe. Diane applies this to her son's mental health issues, but the principles may also be valid for diseases faced by you or your loved ones.

Diane is an early adaptor of a new way of getting well or keeping oneself healthy. Just as my grandfather had no idea what the implications were of the first car he saw driving through his town shortly after the turn of the last century, we also have little idea of the future power of a cooperative relationship between a doctor and an intelligent client using the power of genetic information. What we are seeing now is the Model T and Kitty Hawk airplane stage of genetic computing. This field will change profoundly over the next few years.

Diane's journey is one that is important for anyone with serious health challenges to be aware of and her story may help you in your journey toward optimal health.

- Richard Wilkinson, MD

# Author's Note

———————◆———————

*Never be in a hurry; do everything quietly and in a calm spirit. Do not lose your inner peace for anything whatsoever, even if your whole world seems upset.*
*Saint Francis de Sales*

This is the story of our journey through mental illness and I hope by the end of the book you find a new found hope for yourself and your family members. I was told I should make the telling of the story more flowery, descriptive, and novel like, but truthfully I don't know how to do that from the standpoint of the journey. It wasn't a flowery, novel-like existence; it was a painful, mind numbing, fearful, and solitude building life. So as you read this, you won't feel like you are reading a fictional novel, you will be entering the fragmented, choppy existence that was our life for two decades. Unpacking the trauma in these pages was very difficult and I hope you feel the same things I felt each step of the way. This book reads more like a diary, letting you walk with me through each phase of the journey. I hope you cry with me, get angry with me, and finally find hope in the future with me too.

Mental illness takes a toll on everyone it surrounds. One hard fought lesson I learned is there's always hope, so never give up. It's easy for me to say this now; I wasn't saying it during the almost twenty years of trauma. During our journey, I kept my hope alive by remembering my mentally ill son at a time when he was well and at peace. I held on to snapshots in my mind of our wonderful times together before his illness struck. I held on and remained hopeful for a return to that state sometime in our future.

Writing this book proved to be much more difficult to face than I thought possible; I found I pushed the pain out of my psyche so I could continue to be a wife and mother to my husband and our children over all those years. Dredging up something so few people ever walk through or experience was more emotionally draining than I thought it would be. Recalling the pain and lack of positive progress for so long was overwhelming. I ask myself how anyone survives a mental illness like paranoid schizophrenia. It became apparent to me that we need to give our suffering meaning by how we respond to each other and how we treat one another in the depths of our despair and turmoil, and for this very reason I needed to push forward and finish this book.

It's hard to now realize what Daniel lost during those years of sickness; all the missed opportunities, jobs, life milestones, friends, and romances. Instead he received the alienation of people in the community who didn't understand mental illness. It's a tragedy of epic proportions to see a brilliant young man cut off in his prime with no actual promise for his future. We were told all we could do is medicate, then change the medication every year or two when it no longer worked. It was an aid, it did help with the inability to sleep, but the voices, hallucinations, and delusions remained with him always. There has to be more to this healing than prescription medication, it can't be the only answer.

For all of us out here in the mental illness fight, please try to sit back whenever possible and meditate on the blessings in your life and the hope for a bright future that lays ahead for your family. It's so important to not stay stuck in the negative events, but to clear your head whenever possible. I find myself looking for opportunities to celebrate every fortunate, blessed event in our life.

Through this journey I discovered that our struggles don't define us, our responses to hardships are what shape us and help build our character. The easiest decision would have been to send our child away from our home and change the locks on the door, but we had the freedom to choose and we chose to fight for his life.

I decided to change some of our immediate family names, the physical location where we spent our lives, and most all of the peripheral hospitals, caregivers, facilities, etc. in order to maintain privacy (HIPPA) for all parties involved during this journey. Oregon is a beautiful state and an amazing place to visit. I chose this state at random and with no particular reason in mind.

# Introduction

———————◆———————

*To touch a sore is to renew one's grief.*
*Terence*

Mental illness is something most people turn a blind eye to, cannot understand, or choose not to see, isolating those caught in its grip. We walk a lonely, separate existence, sharing our hurts and burdens with very few people. It's in this solitude that my family lives and breathes. We built our home with love and promises of joy for the future. Our family includes my husband Leonard and myself, our sons Daniel and Tyler, and our daughter Karis. Joys of course do exist, as does a deep abiding love for one another, but at times there's an unwelcome intruder among us, lurking off to the side. It wasn't always this way. We lived in an innocent bubble for fourteen years before our battle with mental illness started. I struggle with where to begin this story of our journey through mental illness and its effect on our family. It so saturates me that most viewpoints during these decades are bleak. Many times in the silence when I'm thinking of our lives, I am overwhelmed with the knowledge that we're blessed to be journeying this tale together, still intact as a family. Some statistics show a divorce rate as high as 80% for couples with a child with disabilities, as compared to the national average of 50%.[iv] Our family holds on and makes the long journey as one.

# Part One

# CHAPTER ONE:

# Here We Go Again – August 2009

———◆———

*Grief can be the garden of compassion. If you keep your heart open through everything, your pain can become your greatest ally in your life's search for love and wisdom.*

*Rumi*

It's summer and Leonard and I are taking our amazing daughter Karis, just out of college, to Washington, D.C., to send her off on a one-year AmeriCorps job. She's volunteering for one year in Minneapolis, Minnesota, in restraining order court. She is going to live with five strangers at poverty level, with no car. These are the parameters of expectation set up within the program. She wants to give back and learn how to live like those less fortunate. Her heart is full of compassion and love. Living with our oldest son who is suffering from mental illness has shaped her and has given her a perspective that no one as young as her should know. It's hard to understand mental illness if it hasn't permeated your very existence. One can read all they want to about mental illness, but walking alongside a sick person gives you a front row seat to the very special and unique pain that so few understand.

It's hard wrapping my mind around letting my daughter go. The daughter that I loved, protected, raised, and sheltered all her life. I can't imagine taking a taxi to the airport to catch my flight and leaving her behind in the hotel room, alone in Washington, D.C., to begin her training before heading off to Minnesota. My husband and I are both struggling. How is this going to work? Leonard is much more excited for her adventure than I am. I'm really going to miss our talks into the night, and our sharing of life and its different nuanced perspectives. I cry silently in the hotel room shower each morning before we go explore Washington, D.C., because I don't want my daughter to see my sadness and grief. Every hour is so painful because it's one hour closer to letting her go. I feel like my heart is going to break. It's so hard to let our children go on to a life they dream about. No one tells you about this separation when you are holding your newborn baby in your arms at the hospital. I've learned you only get to borrow them for a time and then you have to let them go. This is where my mind is when the telephone call comes.

Life changes on a dime, or in this case, on a telephone call. How many telephone calls have I had that changed my life in immeasurable ways? Both of the phone calls letting me know my parents are dead or dying rank up there as life changing and devastating. Over the course of this journey, there have only been a few which fundamentally altered the course of my life as this one does. It's a beautiful day on the sidewalk in Crystal City, Virginia, when my cell phone rings. I answer and it's our middle child, Tyler.

He knows we're in Washington, D.C., but Tyler calls to say, "Bob just called me and I need to go get Daniel because he's really psychotic and can't stay at their apartment any longer." Bob is Daniel's roommate of five years.

Tyler continues, "Daniel's hearing voices and he's afraid of the violent things being said from the people outside their apartment. I guess it's been going on for a while and Bob needs me to come get Daniel because he can't cope with the illness anymore."

Every time I leave town, without fail, Daniel crashes and the phone calls come my way and everything goes into chaos. This time is no different, but the psychosis is more severe and unrelenting. I had no idea he was sliding so far down the rabbit hole. He lives on his own with a roommate, and I'm not always in the loop. I am taken back by the call and wonder what's happening.

Tyler is married with a beautiful wife and two young daughters; he can't bring Daniel to his home while we're gone. I ask Tyler, "Can you please pick up Daniel and take him out to our home and leave him there? I know he'll be alone, but I can't think of anything else we can do right now." I am reasoning that since we live on an acre-and-a-quarter maybe it's secluded enough to keep his bizarre behavior from touching others' lives. I hope Daniel will be okay on his own until I arrive home the next day.

We've been in situations like this before—numerous times—but I have no idea this time will be radically different. After fourteen years, I think I'm getting the hang of taking care of a mentally ill child. But this time, I've no idea the extent of the mental illness with which Daniel is struggling. I have no idea of the anguish, the demons, and the chaotic thoughts that are surrounding my son.

We finish our last day with Karis and go to bed very sober that night wondering what lays ahead for both Karis and Daniel. Leonard and I wake up at the crack of dawn and leave the hotel room with Karis still in her bed wide-awake. She looks so young and innocent lying there watching us pack our bags and getting ready to catch the taxi to the airport. It's a hard separation; I don't want to let her go. But I smile lovingly, tell her just how much I love her and how very proud of her I am. I hug her closely and firmly, cherishing the very smell of her hair. I hold back my tears and act strong as I head out the door after giving her a tight, last hug. I know how blessed I am to have such an amazing daughter. She's such a joy and I am so thrilled to be her momma.

Walking the long hallway of the hotel, I cry quietly, already mourning my lost time with Karis and praying to God that He will keep her safe on this year long journey she is embarking upon. There's one part of me that is so relieved she won't be in Oregon to see the ordeal that lays ahead and that she will not experience the fear and uncertainty of mental illness. She will be safe in Minnesota and won't have to suffer the random bizarre behavior that is taking Daniel over piece by piece.

Leonard and I head out on different flights. Leonard flies off to a worksite down south and I go home alone to Oregon to see what kind of condition Daniel's in and what struggles lay ahead for our family. I choose a seat at my gate where I can look out the window at the tarmac and no one can see me cry silent tears for my daughter. I am also wondering what I'll find at home when I land. Will Daniel be hostile and belligerent, or fragile and shattered? My mind is caught in sadness for Karis, turmoil for Daniel, and I try to breathe…staying calm.

CHAPTER TWO:

# Keep My Son from Torment

———◆———

*To him who is in fear everything rustles.*
*Sophocles*

When I arrive in Oregon and get out to our home, I am stunned to find him in such a fragile, fractured state of mental health. He hasn't slept in days and his eyes are wild, wide open, and glossy. He isn't focusing on much because he's so strung out. He hasn't bathed or done any of the other basic hygiene tasks we all do on a daily basis, and is talking a million miles a minute. "Yesterday people were trying to get into the house, but I wasn't able to catch them, so I called 911 and the police came out. I walked them through the house inside and out and they told me there was nobody in the home and I was safe. I haven't been able to sleep because I can hear people walking around outside the house."

I reassure him, "It's okay, you're not alone now. We'll be just fine. Have you had anything to eat?" I am trying to get him into a calmer state so he can stop pacing so frantically. He's circling the island in the kitchen non-stop, and has been doing this for hours. He can't sit still and he can't be calmed.

After assessing the situation, that evening I call my husband to let him know about Daniel. His paranoia is so pronounced that he can't sleep and he keeps hearing people outside the house threatening him, threatening me, threatening everyone he loves. Unfortunately, Daniel's excessively drinking alcohol and I don't know if he's taking his psychiatric medications. I do know he has a history of stealing pain meds from his roommate and mixing them together, a very lethal combination. At this point in time, we have very little control over his behavior as he is twenty-eight years old. As adults we like to think we control our children, but in Daniel's case our hands are tied by the state. Unfortunately, a mentally ill person has the ability to turn down all care until they're presumed a danger to themselves or to someone else in the community.

While I have Daniel with me at our home, Bob tells me, "A few weeks prior Daniel was standing over my bed while I slept, holding a knife and just staring at me." I am shocked. My mind runs through how horribly this could have ended, with scenario after scenario flicking by in my thoughts.

Bob continues, "I don't believe Daniel would ever do anything to harm me."

"For your own safety, you need to sever the friendship with Daniel until we can get him stable enough so you are truly secure." I'll never forgive myself if something happens to Bob while Daniel is in a psychotic state, thinking God knows what. Bob really struggles with this request as he feels he's abandoning Daniel when he needs him the most.

Bob also lets me know that for the last month or more, he's been covering all the windows in the apartment with blankets because Daniel says there are people outside trying to get in and hurt them. Daniel tells him, "I can hear people outside yelling at the apartment and I'm scared." I am in shock to hear how completely Daniel has lost touch with reality. What seems so simple for me to understand is in fact something Daniel can't grasp. You'd think that by looking out the window you would see no one is there, however, when Daniel looks out, he sees people.

We now have our son living at home with us twenty-four hours a day. Bob follows my wishes and lets Daniel know he isn't going to be able to return to the apartment. After a certain point, it's natural to think things are as bad as they can get, but there's always the potential for worse. I start to realize I need to find inner strength to rise above this perpetual cycle of mental illness. I know I can't control what happens to Daniel and me, but I can control what I do, how I act, and how I feel. When I keep this forefront in my mind I am able to choose how I will respond to the situation. I find I function best when I try and stay logical and calm. It can appear strange to people who are more reactive, but for me I need to do this so I am able to cope with the chaos. I talk to Daniel calmly, and with kindness and compassion. I don't want him to feel judged, found lacking, and blamed for his illness. I measure each word with care so as not to inflict pain and sadness.

As Daniel falls further and further into mental illness, we find him racing to the front door, throwing it open, and looking for the people he hears outside. He does this non-stop for hours and hours and hours, and then days upon days upon days. He's exhausted from trying to catch the people outside who really aren't there. Leonard and I are getting very little sleep because Daniel isn't sleeping due to the voices he's hearing, and the hallucinations he's seeing. One morning around 1 AM, my husband stands in the entry hallway and with his watch he times Daniel to see how often he opens the door trying to catch the people outside. Leonard counts over forty instances in one minute.

He gently tells Daniel, "No one is outside son, you're safe. Please go to bed?" Daniel just can't let it go and is sleeping less and less as the days go by. This of course is causing his psychosis to escalate, and the voices, hallucinations, and delusions are compounding daily.

In another episode, Daniel comes running into the house to get Leonard. "The police are outside and there's a large crowd too. A man is dead in the front yard and the police want to talk to you."

Leonard calmly goes with Daniel and they step out into the yard. No police are here; no dead body is on the ground. All is quiet and the crowd has disappeared. We try to reason with him that these people can't all just disappear so quickly. Daniel insists, "They took the body already, and everyone left. They must have decided they didn't need to discuss the death with you." My husband and I just look at each other in sorrow and dread. Our son is getting worse with each passing week.

During this hard time when Daniel's unraveling, we're also caught up in the fact that he insists he's well. He throws away all of his medication by flushing them down the toilet and refuses to attend his psychiatric appointments. In the past when we've needed help, our usual source was Grace Center, but now Daniel has no psychiatric caregivers at the center as he was kicked out for lack of compliance with their directives. To me, this seems the absolutely worse thing a caregiver can do to a mentally ill person. What do they expect someone who is delusional and caught in a psychosis to do… follow all of their orders?

I contact Daniel's old case manager at Grace and plead with her for help in finding someone she can refer us to who will take care of Daniel's psychiatric needs. She gets him in to a new psychiatrist at New Hope Center in Troutdale. His new psychiatrist is Dr. Patterson and she agrees to care for Daniel. Over the next month, his new doctor begins adjusting his medications on an outpatient basis. She works with us and his new case manager/therapist, Mr. Sonnet, to tweak the meds and dosage. Daniel likes both his new doctor and his new case manager and I'm hopeful this will work.

We spend many days going to New Hope to meet with his new team. I am coordinating my work schedule and making sure Daniel makes each appointment because I can tell he's progressively worsening, even after all of the medication changes. I drive Daniel to his meetings and wait in the intake area for him to talk with his case manager. After they finish talking, the case manager grabs me and we talk about what I see and he gets my take on Daniel's health.

I tell Mr. Sonnet, "I'm not seeing any positive changes. Daniel's lost in a reality that we can't break through." I can tell I am not being heard and they aren't seeing what Leonard and I see at home. I have to wait and let everything play out in its own time.

Unfortunately, their efforts at changing his medications on an outpatient basis and bringing relief to Daniel's psychosis aren't working and his hallucinations continue. I mentioned earlier that you can't just put a person into a mental hospital without him/her being a danger to themselves, or others, but it's true. Your hands are tied when it comes to finding care and being heard. Now I find myself wondering how to work the maze of the psychiatric system to find a way to admit Daniel to the Grace Center Psychiatric Hospital via the emergency room at Providence Medical Center. For me to do otherwise is criminal because Daniel's mental stability is crashing and I need to keep my son from the torment flooding his mind. I worry about the community and everyone's safety. The problem is finding help and a bed where Daniel can receive care.

To do this, you have two choices. One is to go to the crisis response building in Gresham and ring the doorbell in the hopes someone answers and agrees that your loved one needs help. If you ring the doorbell and no one answers, you take your sick loved one home with you or go straight to the emergency room and hope the doctor sees the situation the same way you do. If they agree, they run a drug test to see if the sick person has illegal drugs in their system. If they are drug free, and the doctor agrees there's a problem, then they contact crisis response to come to the emergency room and perform an assessment to see if they also believe a hospital bed is necessary to keep the person or the community safe. Then, of course, a hospital bed needs to be available and open for admission.

There is actually a third option to finding care and that is to contact the police department. I've never taken this approach because of stories I've heard about how the police are not trained to deal with the severely mentally ill, and horrific outcomes can happen. With Daniel so adamant that the government is out to get him and his paranoia of the police, I know that would probably be a recipe for disaster and I don't want to escalate the situation any further.

Unfortunately, within the past two weeks, Daniel and I contacted the crisis response unit by ringing the doorbell at 2 in the morning expressing concern of his decline. The answer is to adjust his medication with his psychiatrist on an outpatient basis as there are no beds available. It's a roller coaster ride as we try to find care.

I thought I'd learned my lesson over the last fourteen years and think I should know how to get care for Daniel. It's frustrating that I'm not successful. I know he needs immediate attention and the only way to ensure I get the mental health community's attention is to arrive at the emergency room and let them see for themselves his mental turmoil. No more doorbell rings late at night at the crisis response unit, to be unanswered, and/or turned away. The problem is Daniel thinks he's fine. I learned that when Daniel is at his sickest, he thinks he's never been better. He won't go with me to the emergency room.

By late August 2009, I contact Daniel's case manager and he tells me to contact crisis response again. Crisis response tells me to take Daniel to Providence Medical Center for a medication clearance test and they'll meet us there to perform an assessment once Daniel's deemed clear of hard narcotics. Now I just pray there's a bed somewhere that we can place Daniel in for immediate care. I think of the crisis response employee, Kathy Little, CDMHP, as my guardian angel. She came to my rescue the last time in the Providence Medical Center emergency room and I'm praying she does the same today. I hope she's the employee who shows up. She knows our history, and she can compare how he's now to how he was last time. She really cares about him and has been helpful in other crisis response visits in the past. Amazingly, it is Ms. Little that arrives and I tell her about Daniel's auditory and visual hallucinations, his internal preoccupation, suicidal ideations, talking about getting a rifle to kill himself, his insomnia which is quite severe, disoriented feelings, hypervigilance, paranoia, and the anxiety that I see in him. His judgment, insight, and impulse control are all grossly impaired. The voices are now giving him commands and occupying all of his time and efforts. He can't shut them off and only recognizes them as real. He's completely internally preoccupied and I can't reach him. No matter how much I talk with him about the people not being real, he's adamant that they're very real. It's amazing to recognize that we've been fighting this war for fourteen long years. Daniel's current diagnosis is Schizoaffective Disorder, Bipolar Type. I keep hope alive by recalling thoughts of Daniel before the illness, and to recognize all of the psychological trauma we've been through and survived so far. I tell myself we'll survive this episode too. It helps me know we'll make it through this.

In the emergency room, Ms. Little finishes the assessment after the medical clearance results comes back clean for narcotics, and the doctors determine Daniel's found safe to be around. The following is her write up and findings:

*"The respondent was brought to Crisis Response today by his mother (Diane Borders (927-xxxx) due to his increasing psychotic symptoms (auditory hallucinations & delusions). The respondent was taken to Providence Medical Center ER for medical clearance prior to CAMHP eval.*

*The respondent has a long (14 year) Hx of suffering with a chronic mental illness (R/O Schizo-affective Disorder) and has had two previous psychiatric hospitalizations at Grace Center. The Respondent is in out-PT services with Dr. Patterson. The respondent has a very supportive mother – who reports that over the past 2-3 weeks the respondent has had increasing auditory hallucinations that he is now responding to – and is having "the voices" tell him to do things (command type) "like to go outside." The respondent's mother, Diane, also reports the respondent has had suicidal ideation at times over the past 2 weeks and has threatened "to get a rifle to kill myself." Evaluated the R @ Providence Medical Center ER. He was cooperative but presents as a somewhat internally preoccupied. The R stated "the voices – I hear are real people" very matter-of-factly. 0x3 stream of thought is clear. Sleep disturbance has become severe (R not slept for almost 24 hours).*

*The respondent's judgment, insight, and impulse control are all grossly impaired. The respondent's O/P provider has already attempted to stabilize the R. on an out PT basis with two recent medication changes – but it has not been successful. No LRA's to in-PT hospitalization are appropriate. The R. is assessed as being a potential danger to self, and also as being gravely disabled due to the increasing severity of his mental illness. The R. is detained involuntarily to Grace Center. Dr. Pershall accepted PT. Providence Amb. Transported."*

Daniel doesn't want to go and is adamant he's fine. I am relieved Kathy sees his illness is escalating, and I'm hopeful this next hospital round will be the one where we land on a prescription drug combination which quiets his mind. We've tried so many different medications and none of them work for long.

He's taken by ambulance from Providence Medical Center to the Grace Center psychiatric hospital. Dr. Namath is the intake psychiatrist who works with Daniel upon admission to the hospital and determines he presents a likelihood of serious harm to himself and is gravely disabled. He prescribes Risperdal and Zyprexa Zydis for control of his psychotic symptoms, Lithium for mood stabilization, and Valium for anxiety. I am praying the new medication, Zyprexa Zydis, will work, but how often have I prayed this prayer? I know new medications are in the pipeline for mental illness, but they can't get here soon enough. I often think to myself that there has to be some other answer to mental illness than just medicating the symptoms away with a prescription drug. I remember hearing a saying "Don't quit five minutes before the miracle happens" and I think of this often and hope things will be different this time. We've tried so many prescription drugs for Daniel's mental illness and none of them worked, there are very few drugs we haven't tried. I feel at a loss for where to turn next if this hospitalization doesn't come up with a new drug combination that alleviates the voices, hallucinations, and delusions.

As I sit thinking into the night, I start to wonder about the most basic unit of our health, which I believe is cell function. I often find myself wondering what's wrong on the cellular level within Daniel's body. I've been researching genetic mutations and am starting to believe this has to play a role in his wellbeing. There are genetic mutations in our body which affect many biochemical processes that need to be working correctly in order for us to have health. Genetic mutations called single nucleotide polymorphisms are a new field of study. What little I've found in research is so cutting edge most doctors don't know what to do with the questions I ask, or even where to turn for answers. But I also think, "We don't have genetic mutations. After all, aren't people with genetic mutations really ill?"

During this hospitalization, Dr. Namath lets us know Daniel may be transferred to another inpatient facility if the treating physician decides it's necessary – meaning he presents a likelihood of serious harm to himself, serious harm to others, or is gravely disabled. The only other inpatient facility I can think of is the state mental hospital at Medford. As I sit here and listen, I wonder why didn't his doctor and case manager try to get him hospitalized earlier; why did I have to fight so hard? Why is everything such a battle? It's not like I have a huge reservoir of energy.

We have a new doctor assigned to Daniel during this hospitalization. His name is Dr. Charles Egan. During this hospital stay, Daniel's quiet and withdrawn. When we sit with him in the evening during visiting hours, he's guarded and makes paranoid statements. He believes people are trying to harm him and his sleep is poor; he can't seem to turn off his mind, the voices, and their messages.

Dr. Egan tells us Daniel is compliant with taking his medications as asked. He spends time with Daniel each day and learns that Daniel believes he's empowered by a demon named Loci, and he invites Loci to give him guidance every day. Daniel lets the doctor know, "All of the good in my life comes from Loci who gives me commands." Dr. Egan plans to use the demon Loci to his advantage to open Daniel up to the inner strength that Daniel has innately. I can't wrap my mind around this logic, it doesn't even make sense. I don't even know what the doctor is saying…it sounds crazy. He seems to think he can twist the power of Loci and morph it into integrating Daniel into one whole being. Huh?

Dr. Egan also tells me, "I learned that Daniel believes his dad loves him, but you do not." In digging further into this thought process, the doctor finds out he believes in his twisted mind that he can manipulate and influence his dad to have sex with him. He doesn't believe he can influence me to have sex with him, so therefore, I don't love him. Leonard and I sit there dumbfounded as the doctor enlightens us to Daniel's thinking. We're both in shock to hear the distorted thought process inside his mind and I can see just how far Daniel has fallen under the spell of his voices and delusions.

According to the psychiatric team, Daniel continues to take his medication as prescribed and he's now participating in their treatment program. He still has periods of anxiety and his affect (external expression of emotions) remains blunted, but he's showing improvement and they believe he's stabilizing. Near the end of the fourteen days of inpatient treatment, Daniel is interviewed by legal representatives from the state and his psychiatric team for the purpose of a Least Restrictive Alternative (LRA) agreement hearing, and he's calm and appropriate. The LRA is all about the ability to involuntarily hold a mentally ill patient (civil commitment) if they're not following certain guidelines as specified in the agreement, as determined necessary by the physician and the courts. The mental health community wants to hold the mentally ill person in a manner which is least restrictive to their ability to get around and be free. Therefore, they just need to abide by certain rules and restrictions as drawn up in the LRA. There are fourteen, ninety, and one hundred eighty day LRAs.

The petition for revocation of less restrictive alternative agreement reads as follows:

*"The respondent is a 28-year-old, single, Caucasian male who resides in Portland, Oregon. He has a history of mental illness with two prior inpatient psychiatric hospitalizations. He was enrolled in outpatient mental health services at New Hope Counseling Center in Troutdale, Oregon prior to his admission.*

*The respondent was detained at Grace Center on August 27, 2009. His mother had contacted the Crisis Response Unit (CRU) on several occasions over the previous two weeks, expressing concern that the respondent was deteriorating. Attempts were made by the respondent's outpatient providers to adjust his medication, but his symptoms continued to increase. The respondent was brought to CRU on the day of his detention.*

*His mother reported he had experienced increased auditory hallucinations, delusions and decreased sleep. He had reported increasing suicidal ideations over the previous two weeks and the attempts to adjust his medication were unsuccessful. The respondent was taken to Providence Medical Center and evaluated by a DMHP after he was medically cleared. According to the detention documents the respondent had threatened to kill himself by using a rifle. His sleep was poor and he hadn't slept in 24 hours. His insight judgment and impulse control were impaired and he was detained as a danger to self and gravely disabled.*

*Upon admission to Grace Center the respondent was described as quiet and withdrawn. He was guarded at times and made paranoid statements, believing people were trying to harm him. His sleep remained poor, but he was compliant with taking his medications as prescribed. He appeared to be responding to internal stimuli and experienced periods of response latency. He was committed for up to 14 more days on September 1, 2009. While at Grace Center the respondent has continued to take medication as prescribed and participates in the treatment program. He continues with periods of anxiety and his affect remains blunted, but he has shown improvement and is stabilizing.*

*The respondent was interviewed for the purpose of a hearing and informed of his rights on September 10, 2009. He agreed to be interviewed. He was calm and appropriate. He denied suicidal or homicidal ideations. He reports his sleep has improved and denied side effects from the medication. He denied auditory hallucinations at the time of this interview and reports he believes he is stable and ready for discharge. The treatment team believes the respondent is nearing his baseline functioning and is ready for discharge. It is recommended he be released on an LRA. The structure and support of the LRA will help ensure the respondent remains in services and stable in the community."*

Daniel's released from Grace Center on the following medication: Risperdal, Lithium, Effexor, Melatonin, Zebeta and Iron. I know this is a sham and he's no better, but all the psychiatric team members seem to think he's good to go, so Daniel is released. Family members aren't asked what they see, what was said to them by the patient during the stay, or what they think about the stability of their loved ones. We who are responsible for their care aren't asked anything. If Leonard or I were included, we could tell them about things we saw as we visited Daniel each evening while he was inpatient. If this new doctor and the hospital staff think he has reached his baseline of normalcy, then we're all in big trouble. Daniel knows what the doctor and staff want to hear, and he wants out. He feels he isn't sick, and the voices are more real than the physical people surrounding him. But, Daniel knows he has to deny their existence and he tells the doctor and staff what they want to hear. He says he'll comply and he responds however he needs to in order to be free and out of the facility.

Daniel is released into the care of his new doctor along with a new case manager. The new psychiatric team is from Grace Center where he has been under their care before during the last fifteen years. Hopefully, this time he won't get kicked out of their care for non-compliance of the requirements of his LRA. I'm always hopeful at every change that this new psychiatric team will have some new insight and new ideas to try to bring Daniel back to sanity.

He returns to the apartment he shares with Bob. Unfortunately, as I expect, he immediately starts drinking alcohol to excess, and he does not comply with his medications as if the hospitalization and the legal proceedings were a joke. I feel terrible that Bob is having to deal with Daniel's behavior, and I marvel at Bob's patience for his antics. I don't know what to do and I am frustrated at the entire system. It's like a bad dream I can't escape.

One month later in early October 2009, I let Daniel's new case manager, Peggy Nicks-Keller, know he's drinking heavily, a violation of his LRA. His alcohol consumption is up to thirty-two cans of beer within an hour or two, followed by blacking out. He'll do anything to get alcohol, including stealing money from his family and friends. His case manager doesn't do anything with the information even though I stress this is breaking his LRA. I don't get a response and I feel like I'm the only one trying to keep him alive. His LRA is meaningless because the psychiatric team doesn't enforce the document.

During the month, I attend a one-day conference held by Dr. Daniel Amen who talks about his new technology which studies the brains of ill people using Single-Photon Emission Computerized Tomography (SPECT) scans.[v] Using these scans, he can tell just what kind of medication the brain needs to function adequately. I know at this point, Daniel is too sick for me to have a rational, productive conversation with him about this new technology, but I decide I will talk to him when we hit a point where he's well enough to understand. The technology sounds promising and I'm always researching options out in the scientific community that might benefit my son. He needs to be off all psychiatric medications in order to have the SPECT scan done, and I'm not sure how we'll ever make that happen because he's so sick.

There are times when his roommate lets me know I need to come get Daniel, or Bob drops him off at our home on his way to work. As Daniel decompensates, Bob can't handle him anymore and is afraid he'll be kicked out of his apartment due to Daniel's behavior. At one point, Bob brings Daniel to us and asks us to care for him. My husband and I limp along with him drinking and not taking his medications. Not surprisingly he's caught up in a few delusions which totally encompass his waking thoughts.

Daniel informs me, "I was selected as the winner of the America's Next Top Model competition." He's talking a million miles a minute, and he's so excited for the honor. I sit in shock at his statement, but smile at him and ask him for more information. He tells me, "They're coming in a limousine on Friday at 5 PM to pick me up and take me to a taping at the television station." Finally, I think, this one will be easy to disprove because there will be no limo showing up on Friday at 5 PM. It's amazing what his brain can do to his reality.

So we wait. Daniel is really excited as the day approaches; he's up in the bathroom grooming himself in preparation of the arrival of the America's Next Top Model team. He comes down the stairs with his hair heavily coated in some kind of gel, actually dripping wet with product. As evening arrives, he and I wait in the formal living room, anticipating the doorbell. Five o'clock comes and goes, and no one is at the door. Daniel goes off into the bathroom and when he comes back I think now is a good time to discuss the delusion. I broach the subject that the whole thing is a delusion and it never happened.

He looks at me, "Oh no, they called me and said they have to delay it for a week due to scheduling changes."

This is when I realize no matter how many hard facts I have on my side, or how blatant the delusion is, his mind will always have a reason for any change, and this is his brain protecting itself. I am speechless and I have no comeback. It takes some processing of my own to realize I can't fight his delusions because I can never win the discussion.

During the past two weeks, Daniel's been telling me, "I want to commit suicide, I'm tired of this, and I want it to all be over with." He's fixated on death and wanting this life to be done. I'm sitting in his room trying to talk to him.

"If you will just take your medications," I tell him, "if you will stop drinking alcohol, if you will begin eating a normal diet and get adequate nutrition, you'll start to feel better." It seems like I just keep saying, if, if, if…and he never takes me up on any of the suggestions which might improve the chances of his medication working.

Things are getting so bad I'm truly afraid he'll die before I can get anyone to respond with any action to save him. I mean real action, not a silly in-and-out revolving door of the psychiatric hospital. After all, didn't the doctors just release him from the mental hospital a few weeks ago? I know he's sick even though they released him out into the public, but with the courts and physicians all in favor of keeping the sick, mentally ill people out in the community, there isn't much power in the family member's call for help.

# CHAPTER THREE:

## Keep My Son Alive and Breathing

———◆———

*Shall I tell you what the real evil is? To cringe to the things that are called evils, to surrender to them our freedom, in defiance of which we ought to face any suffering.*
*Lucius Annaeus Seneca*

During the month of October 2009, things go downhill even more rapidly. When Daniel has the opportunity to talk with me alone, he says such horrifying things for my ears only. He tells me, "I want to bludgeon blondes with a baseball bat. I think about it all the time." How does a mom even respond to a comment like that? I stuff my response and don't say anything, but it makes me afraid for the community. I have blonde hair and I wonder if I am the target of the voices and delusions. My daughter-in-law is blonde, as are both of my granddaughters. Of course, because of this comment, Tyler won't allow his family to be around Daniel unless I'm in the same space.

I immediately call the case manager and let her know about his comment. I tell her my fears about our home being on a public walking path where children ride bicycles and fish in the pond. Daniel sits out on the patio and smokes, all the while watching the path. I can't imagine the agony if anything happened. It doesn't seem to cause concern with the case manager, and no action is taken. I guess this is the part where Daniel has to cause harm to himself or the community before action is taken. I make sure the case manager knows I'm on record with them about the fantasies.

In late October, Daniel is back living at the apartment with Bob. I am relieved because he's no longer at our home, and he's no longer able to sit and watch the walking path. One evening as I'm leaving work, I get a phone call from Bob. He asks me, "Will you please go to my apartment. Daniel's been drinking for three days straight with no sleep. He just stole money from me and went to the store to purchase a case and a half of beer. He drank all of the beer in a very short time and passed out." Bob also thinks he took a bunch of Valium because he found the bottle empty and some of the pills scattered on the floor in the living room beside Daniel.

In contemplative worry he says, "There was probably little more than a half month's supply of pills in the bottle of Valium before Daniel got ahold of it." He takes a breath before continuing, "I really need to get to work so I am not fired, and I'm afraid Daniel will die while I am at work. I need you to stop over at our apartment to make sure Daniel is still alive. I am leaving the sliding glass door unlocked for you so you can enter the apartment to check on him." And he hangs up.

I head over to their apartment after work with a heavy heart, expecting to find the worse possible scenario. I let myself in through the slider and find Daniel in the living room, lying on the ground face down beside the sofa, totally unresponsive. I feel his neck for his carotid artery and check to see if his heart is beating. Thank God, he's alive, but his breathing is shallow. I know he needs help soon because the next time he may die from this lethal combination. I also know it'll do me no good to reach out to his psychiatric team who've been unresponsive so far, so I leave the apartment and head home with a really worried mind.

I call Bob and let him know, "Daniel's breathing with a shallow pulse." I won't lie… a part of me thought this might be an easy way for Daniel to pass away. If Daniel didn't wake up, his troubles would be over and his pain and suffering would be done. I remember all of the times I told Daniel to hold on, there was something in the future that would bring relief. We can't ever let that thought go, otherwise this existence would be unbearable. I find myself praying for God to keep my son alive until I can get someone, anyone, to respond and give us help.

The next morning, October 29, 2009, I again phone Daniel's case manager at the Grace Center to let her know what happened last evening. This time she contacts the crisis response unit and talks to Kathy Little, CDMHP, to tell her about the events of the night before. She lets Kathy know Daniel violated every condition of his LRA.

Kathy calls me and asks me, "Is he still in the apartment?"

"According to Bob, he is."

Kathy contacts the Gresham police to let them know a 'detain and transfer' order is signed, and she goes to meet the police at Bob's apartment.

Kathy waits in her car outside the apartment as the police head in to talk with Daniel. I am on the phone with Kathy as the police approach the apartment. I know how bad these situations can go when mentally ill people are confronted by the police. Daniel has a fear of the police and the government and I'm praying God will keep my son calm, subdued, and compliant. I hope everything goes smoothly when they knock on the apartment door and I'm terrified the outcome will quickly turn bad. I am sitting in the ladies' restroom at work because this is the only place where my cell phone gets any reception. I am trying to keep it together as my coworkers come in and out, but I end up softly crying as the events play out. Kathy gives me a blow by blow account of the movements of the police. I feel relief to know they recognize they're dealing with a mentally ill patient and the mental health worker knows Daniel and can apprise them of his mental state. The police knock on the apartment door, and Daniel answers.

"Daniel's acknowledging to the police the level of alcohol and pills from the night before. He knows this breaks his LRA which is a condition of his release from the mental hospital during his inpatient stay last month." Kathy relays.

I am starting to be able to breathe again, and I'm less afraid of violence occurring as each minute passes. I am so relieved because I know with him breaking the agreement, he'll go back to inpatient care and they'll adjust his medication, maybe hit on a new combination that will help.

The police take Daniel to the Gresham hospital where they perform a medical clearance test. Once he clears the test, Kathy is able to assess him. I hurry over to the hospital to be there when the police drop Daniel off, and to talk to Kathy. Again, she'll be the person who listens, responds, and gives me help. I truly think of her as my touchstone in the fight for Daniel.

I tell her, "He's becoming increasingly hostile to me and texting me messages to 'fuck off' and other crude things." I show the text messages to Kathy and let her know, "This isn't his normal behavior, it's escalating."

With a voice that begins to tremble, I also tell her, "He's calling me in the night and leaving ranting, hate filled, incoherent ramblings. I've been turning off my phone at night so I can sleep without being hit with these calls." I solemnly tell her, my eyes downcast in sorrow.

In the emergency room, Daniel appears to be internally preoccupied and he tells Kathy, "I'm America's Next Top Model." He's lying on the hospital bed, and comes in and out of it with disjointed comments about being a model, and being on TV. Daniel's judgment, insight, and impulse control are all impaired and this is very apparent to Kathy. She requests the ninety-day LRA be revoked and she detains Daniel involuntarily for re-stabilization on his medications. No LRA is available at this time as Daniel is a danger to himself or others. He's taken to the Grace Center hospital again.

Dr. Egan talks with Daniel and I find out that Daniel quit his medication over two weeks ago. He also missed his mental health appointments with both his case manager and his psychiatrist, and he's abusing alcohol. He's responding to auditory hallucinations and Dr. Egan tells us Daniel is "talking to Satan." As the days' progress at the hospital I find out that the night I went in through the slider at Bob's apartment to check on Daniel that he'd taken ten to twelve Valium pills and had been drinking heavily because he couldn't fall asleep.

One evening during this hospital stay, Leonard and I arrive to see Daniel together because I can't be alone with him as he now believes I am a problem. He is very hostile to me. A nurse approaches me to let me know that Daniel picked up the phone at the nurses' station and called 911. When the operator picked up, he told her that he was in the hospital and there was a fight going on in the parking lot.

She continues, "When the inpatient nurse approached him to ask what he was doing, he told her he was letting the police know there was a fight taking place outside the hospital. He's hearing voices outside the facility non-stop and he's so preoccupied with listening to the voices over the wall that no one can get him to talk or focus on anything."

It's heartbreaking to watch his mind failing him. The hospital starts Daniel on Invega Sustenna IM injections once a month. The other medications they place him on are Antabuse and Melatonin at night. The addition of Antabuse is a new part of his LRA which will be a requirement for his upcoming release. According to the doctor, the Antabuse will make him extremely, deathly ill if he drinks alcohol while taking this medication. Daniel promises he won't drink and he's willing to take the Antabuse. Another aspect of this new LRA is that Daniel needs to attend a substance abuse assessment at the Mentally Ill/Chemically Addicted (MICA) program.

"I am becoming increasingly frightened of Daniel and I'm not comfortable with him living in our home," I tell Dr. Egan. The medical team sends an application to the Connor House, and Daniel is handed an application to the Onyx House. The Onyx House is a home that expects residents to meet certain specific expectations. I don't believe Daniel will be accepted because he won't follow even the most basic rules. The voices drive him to feel he knows better than other people and he follows them to the exclusion of all else. Daniel has stayed at the Connor House a couple times in the past and they also have rules the patients need to follow and curfews to respect. During past stays Daniel and the other residents bought or stole beer and hide it behind the shed in the backyard. When the patients went out to smoke, they grabbed the hidden beer and drank it in the dark. It's amazing how much alcohol addiction drives them to get beer, no matter what the cost. I'm nervous about how Daniel will respond to drinking alcohol and having it mix with Antabuse. I know he'll drink no matter what he tells his psychiatric team. He's a great manipulator and can appear so convincingly normal. I know better because I'm always left cleaning up the mess when the doctors discharge him back in the community.

Daniel's assigned a new case manager, Karen Everett, during this hospital stay. He's still working with Dr. Egan who continues to follow his plan of integrating Daniel's voices, and the demon Loci, into one within him. I am hesitant about this idea because I'm the focal point of all his aggression and vulnerable if he follows through on the things he says he wants to do. Not only that, but I have no protection when they let him out. It's easy for the doctors and staff to say they want to do this thing or that thing when they are safely home, not living with the threat of harm.

Daniel receives a Notice of Potential Loss of Firearm Rights in the mail. In this instance, his failure to seek voluntary treatment and subsequent detention for involuntary treatment results in the loss of his right to possess a firearm. He doesn't own a firearm and doesn't have any money to his name to purchase one, but it's nice to know that some paperwork trails for the mentally ill are working. But there are other ways to kill or injure people. Fewer than 5% of mentally ill people killed with guns from 2000 to 2009.[vi] However, another study showed that being in high risk relationships give you an 85% chance of being killed by a gun if the person is within your social network.[vii] At this point, knives and baseball bats seem to be the weapon of choice for Daniel in his delusions, but you never know where the voices and delusions will take him.

Upon discharge from this hospital stay on November 16, 2009, Daniel is living at our home again because he's becoming more and more out of control and isn't able to stay with Bob. Even suggesting his discharge is ridiculous. How can Daniel be released out into the community when his roommate can't even allow him to come back to their apartment? Something is wrong with our mental health system if he's well enough to be released but not well enough for his roommate to allow him to stay with him at the apartment. Because of this we have the mentally ill out on the streets and homeless with no care for even their most basic needs. We aren't doing our mentally ill a service by the laws and the system as regulated.

Upon his discharge we find out his insurance won't pay for Invega Sustenna due to the cost. As long as he's hospitalized they'll cover the cost of the once a month injection, but upon his release, it's no longer covered. This makes no sense. Who comes up with these rules? Instead, Daniel is approved for the Consta IM injection every two weeks. It's the same medication, it just doesn't last as long so compliance is harder to maintain for the patient. The Invega Sustenna IM long acting injections are stopped after just two doses which are administered while Daniel is inpatient. Each time they change his medication I am hopeful they'll work better and longer, but they never do the job. I pray for Daniel to be responsive to these new medications so he can find peace from the voices.

On November 30, 2009, in the state superior court, the petition for an extension on Daniel's LRA reads as follows:

*"The respondent is a 28-year-old, single, Caucasian male who resides in Portland, Oregon. He is currently in outpatient mental health services with Grace Center under a court order which is set to expire on December 14, 2009.*

*The respondent has a history of mental illness and has previous psychiatric hospitalizations. He has had two involuntary hospitalizations within the last three months. The respondent had initially been hospitalized on August 28th, 2009, after being evaluated as gravely disabled and danger to self. He was treated at Grace Center inpatient unit until his discharge on September 15th, 2009 under a 90-day outpatient court order. However, the respondent was re-detained on October 29th, 2009, after the respondent's case manager contacted Crisis Response Unit reporting that the respondent has violated all the conditions of his LRA and was decompensating. The respondent had reportedly missed all but one of his mental health appointments since his discharge from Grace Center. The respondent had discontinued taking medication after his prescription ran out and made no effort to refill the medication. His family reported that the he had become increasingly hostile towards them and appeared to be responding to internal stimuli. His insight, judgment, and impulse control were all described as impaired and he was admitted again to Grace Center inpatient unit for emergency treatment.*

*At this time the treatment team is endorsing an extension of the respondent's LRA. According to the treatment team, the respondent continues to present with symptoms of a mental illness and requires ongoing support to remain in the community. By report, the respondent presents with depression and at times is latent response. The treatment team has placed the respondent on injectable medication due to issues with oral medication compliance. The treatment team does not believe that the respondent would continue treatment in good faith as a voluntary patient at this time. Additional extension of the respondent's court ordered treatment plan is recommended to be in his best interest at this time."*

I appreciate the staff staying on top of Daniel's LRA and keeping it active in case we need the ability to pull him back into psychiatric care. It's truly only a matter of time. By Daniel's demeanor, I know it's not over by any means.

Pretty quickly after his discharge, Daniel's stealing alcohol and coming home and drinking until he blacks out. Amazingly, he's doing this while on Antabuse. I thought the combination of Antabuse and alcohol was deadly, but apparently not for Daniel. I talk to my boss, Pam, about the situation, and she's saddened as she was the first person to give Daniel a job while he was in high school; he means a lot to her and her family. She volunteers to come with me when I find out that he's at our home, and quite drunk. He isn't throwing up on the Antabuse and he isn't sick in any other way except his skin is turning really bright red. He's lying on his bed and sobbing, "I want this life to be over with…I'm so tired."

He wants to commit suicide to find peace. He can't let this thought go. Life is just too hard to bear. I contact Daniel's new case manager to let her know.

"He's violating his LRA once again and he's drinking while on Antabuse, and talking about suicide."

She's amazing and immediately jumps into action to help me with Daniel. I can tell I have a winner in this new case manager, so different from most all of the responses in the past.

On December 9, 2009, Ms. Everett takes Daniel to the Detox Unit. It's the evening of my office Christmas party but there's no holiday joy this year. We are sitting at my company's dinner party and we can't get into the spirit of the holidays, so my husband and I leave the Christmas dinner early and go to the detox facility. Daniel is disoriented and lost. When we arrive the staff tells us Daniel stripped naked and was yelling profanities. They can't get him to keep his clothes on and he's not coherent. The facility determines it's not safe for him to reenter the community. They detain him and will watch him as he sobers up in case there are dangerous alcohol withdrawal symptoms.

Daniel's had a few detox stints at this facility and each time he's released with the stipulation that he must attend a dual diagnosis program to work on the addiction and the mental illness combination. A dual diagnosis program is for the mentally ill who also have another factor affecting their ability to be treated, such as drug addiction or alcoholism. So far, he always says, "I don't need it, it's not useful," and stops attending.

During this stay at the detox facility, Daniel is found quite intoxicated and reporting homicidal ideations. One day, the detention staff at the center contact crisis response reporting he's becoming increasingly psychotic and difficult to manage. They request an Involuntary Treatment Act (ITA) evaluation. According to the detox detention documents, Daniel hasn't slept and is becoming increasingly agitated. They observe him yelling, using profanity, and disturbing other clients. He requires several redirections from the staff for wandering around the facility naked. They observe him talking to himself and repeatedly looking over his shoulder, appearing to be responding to internal stimuli. The staff at the detox center indicates they're no longer able to manage his symptoms, and they note that my husband and I don't feel we can keep our son safe. They detain him as gravely disabled. On December 14, 2009, the detox facility decides Daniel's too sick to keep in their building and they move him to the Grace Center hospital. They let the case manager know he's gravely mentally ill and they aren't equipped to care for him. This is his third inpatient stay in three months.

While in the mental hospital during the month of December, Daniel calls 911 from the nurses' station, saying, "I'm being tortured." The nurses have to keep a close eye on him because he's preoccupied with the people in his hallucinations to the detriment of everything else. He truly has no grasp on reality and this psychotic state is overpowering and very real to him. The nurse pulls me to the side to let me know about this phone call and how lost he is in his own reality. It's good to have the staff willing to give me updates on how he's doing. It makes me feel calm as I leave after the visit knowing eyes are being kept on him to ensure he stays safe.

While Daniel is at the Grace Center, he's complying with staff requests but he still remains symptomatic. The staff make note of his confusion and restlessness. His affect is flat, again not reacting in a normal way to his surroundings, and he continues to appear to be responding to internal stimuli. His appetite is poor and he won't eat. They say he has bizarre thoughts of killing and eating people. He's mumbling to himself constantly, talking to himself one moment and then laughing at what he perceives to be funny statements coming from his hallucinations.

Dr. Egan orders Risperdal Consta (atypical antipsychotic) injections because it is a longer duration medication for hallucinations and psychosis. This helps because we're always trying to ensure every day medication compliance. They monitor the effectiveness of the injections during their daily sessions. Dr. Egan plans to use intervention to assist Daniel to understand his negative thoughts, to assess Daniel's mood in daily sessions, and administer interventions related to his issues for alcohol abuse, mood, and safety. Dr. Egan also assists Daniel with a search for MICA inpatient treatment and referral program, along with planning doctor appointments up to two times a week, within seven days of his discharge.

Unfortunately, during the stay Daniel's found to have high thyroid levels in his blood work and he has a scan of the thyroid done. They say he has hyperthyroidism which causes the thyroid gland to produce excess thyroid hormone. This condition can cause many different health problems such as a rapid heart rate, weight loss, trouble sleeping, fatigue, nervousness and anxiety. Daniel's taken off Invega Consta injections because Dr. Egan believes it's affecting his thyroid. Now we're back to hoping we can get Daniel to comply with taking his pills. I sit there listening to the doctor wondering if there isn't something else we can do to help his thyroid, while still allowing him to take the Invega Consta injections. At least that way we wouldn't have to worry about him swallowing pills every day and being noncompliant on his medication management.

An LRA is initiated for one hundred eighty days (6 months) effective December 14, 2009. In the superior court of the state of Oregon in and for the county of Multnomah, the petition for revocation of the LRA reads as follows:

*"The respondent is a 28-year-old, single, Caucasian male who resides in Portland, Oregon with his parents. He has a history of mental illness and prior inpatient psychiatric hospitalizations. He received outpatient mental health services at Grace Center and is monitored on a 180-day LRA that has been entered earlier on the day of this detention. The respondent was detained to Grace Center on December 14, 2009.*

*The respondent was placed in the detox center on December 9, 2009 after violating the terms of his LRA and becoming intoxicated and reporting homicidal ideations. The day of his detention staff at the detox center contacted Crisis Response Unit (CRU) reporting the respondent was becoming increasingly psychotic and difficult to manage. An ITA evaluation was requested. According to the detention documents the respondent had not slept the night before and was becoming increasingly agitated. He was observed yelling and using profanity, disturbing other clients. He required several redirections from the staff for wandering around the facility naked. He was observed talking to himself and repeatedly looking over his shoulder, appearing to be responding to internal stimuli. Staff at the detox center indicated they were no longer able to manage his symptoms and his parents did not feel they could keep the respondent safe. He was detained as gravely disabled.*

*While at Grace Center the respondent has complied with staff requests, but remains symptomatic. He presents with confusion and restlessness. His affect is described as flat and he continues to appear to be responding to internal stimuli.*

*His appetite remains poor and he required redirection for calling 911 to report he was being tortured.*

*The respondent was interviewed for the purpose of a hearing and informed of his rights on December 17, 2009. He agreed to be interviewed. The respondent was guarded when questioned about the events leading to the detention, but indicated he has felt fatigued and confused at times. He admitted to recent alcohol use and acknowledged it violated the conditions of his LRA. He also reported homicidal ideations, but attributed these feelings to his alcohol consumption. He reported he called 911 while at Grace Center because he felt he was being psychologically tortured by his ex-girlfriend believing she was accusing him of being a sex offender. When questioned if he had spoken to his ex-girlfriend recently he denied and then gave a disorganized explanation of why he felt this way, eventually stating he thinks he may be paranoid. The treatment team believes the respondent is in need of further inpatient treatment for medication stabilization and discharge planning. He violated the conditions of his LRA and it is recommended the order be revoked for up to the remainder of the 180-days."*

The next week passes with the inpatient team trying to stabilize Daniel on medication. So far I'm not seeing any change in his state. It seems like we've tried every medication on the market. It all just seems so hopeless. However, we decide to check him out of the hospital for a four-hour visit on Christmas Day. We want him with us knowing he's still an important, crucial part of our family and we haven't turned our backs on him in his illness. It isn't easy having him with us during the day, and it is tense, but he spends most of his time pacing in circles out in the driveway, laughing and talking to himself, totally disconnected from our family.

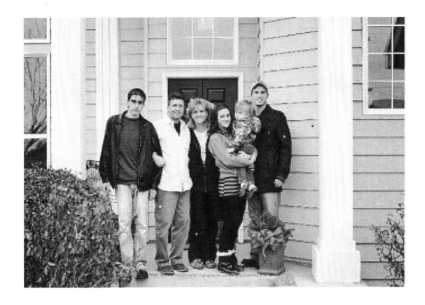

On December 27, 2009, Dr. Egan states the following in regards to Daniel:

*"Patient has a history of Schizo affective disorder. He was just recently readmitted to the hospital due to medication noncompliance and also alcohol abuse. When he abuses substances he decompensates rather quickly. Patient needs help from case management. He has poor insight into his illness. He needs to be continued on an LRA so that he can comply with treatment and stay safe in the community."*

On January 5, 2010, Daniel is discharged from the Grace Center on a LRA. Medications upon release are Abilify (2 mg/day) and melatonin (10 mg) at bedtime. Dr. Egan states he'll work with Daniel to integrate the voices into one person within Daniel. He has a follow up appointment with his case manager, and Sharon Watts, medication management. Daniel should see an Endocrinologist for his abnormal thyroid results. A referral to Passages in Redmond for inpatient mental illness/chemical addiction (MICA) treatment program is issued.

My first gut reaction to his release isn't favorable. Here we go again. How can Daniel function on just Abilify and melatonin if he has the diagnosis of schizoaffective disorder, bipolar type? I know in my heart this is a grave under-medication for Daniel. He's going to slip further into psychosis and our family is going to be stuck scrambling for safety and help. How can the doctor believe Abilify is a safe alternative to injectable anti-psychotics? How can healthcare coverage pay for an injectable anti-psychotic that lasts for a month while in the hospital, and then say, "Oh no coverage, if you are discharged as stable and safe for the community"? How do they think the patient became stable? Wasn't it the injectable that got them there? Why then would you no longer cover the same medication on an outpatient basis? It's like every step of the way you're set up for hardship and disaster. I find my anger and fury building after each subsequent inpatient hospital stay and discharge. I'm beginning to think I need to find the answer myself because our state and government systems are ineffective in almost every area. I hope our family stays safe, and protected against what's being unleashed back into our home.

The doctor brings me in to see him and visits with me prior to Daniel's release to let me know they'll actively pursue a spot in a mental illness/chemical addiction treatment program (MICA/dual diagnosis program).

"I'm anxious and scared to have Daniel living with us in our home because I know he won't comply, no matter what he tells you. We're the ones left to try and pick up the pieces of his shattered mind." I tell the doctor, "We live on a public walking path right at the end of our backyard. Daniel sits out back smoking and can see children and adults from the community walk by throughout the day. If the voices are able to convince him to act, there may be huge consequences for the public."

I make sure I'm on record stating this fact in case something horrible happens. Often times, when a family member harms someone in the community, the community wants to find the family and lay the blame at their feet. They ask, "Why didn't you get the person help?" They just don't realize no matter how hard the family tries, there isn't help to be found much of the time. Resources are spread too thin, funding isn't allocated, and beds are too few and far between. Unfortunately, our state and federal systems don't adequately fund mental health care. We spend our precious tax dollars on the worried well, not the severely mentally ill. We need to rethink the way we spend our tax dollars and care for the mentally ill who are falling through the cracks and ending up on the streets.

I leave work on the morning of January 5, 2010, when they release Daniel and pick him up from the Grace Center hospital, trying to put on a positive face. I am hoping by stuffing my anxiety, I'm showing a countenance of hope. Daniel seems calm as we head to our home. On the way we swing by and pick up his Abilify medication. We haven't tried this medicine before, so as usual I'm hopeful this may work.

Three days later, on January 8, Daniel is accepted into the Passages program. It's a six-week outpatient treatment program to work on addiction in the presence of mental illness. I'm hopeful this program will have better luck than the MICA program. On the morning of January 8, I wake Daniel up and head to Passages. His first three days are spent at a Redmond detox facility, a customary procedure. After completing the detox, they move him to Passages on Monday. I get a phone call on Friday morning, four days after Daniel starts Passages, and they tell me, "Come and get him because he won't participate in the program or take his medicine. He refuses to get out of bed and won't talk to anyone." Passages tells me they believe something is wrong with his health, and I think, "No kidding."

I'm in shock when they tell me to just come pick him up. Isn't he violating his LRA? Shouldn't he be put back into the mental hospital for noncompliance of this legal order? Why are his doctor, case manager, and medications nurse, just turning a blind eye to his expulsion from Passages? I'm so frustrated that the system is so fractured. How is someone supposed to get help for their sick loved one when there's no way to force the treatment that will supposedly bring the help? When I arrive at Passages, I ask them these questions and they tell me, "There are so many people in need of our beds that if a person won't cooperate, they're kicked out of the facility."

I start to cry when I tell them, "You are pushing out a severely ill young man who needs your help and is too sick to know any better."

"Sorry," they reply, "There's nothing we can do to help you or your son."

We're living in a bubble made up of fractured, unkept promises. Daniel will say all the right things to his psychiatric team and he easily manipulates them to his benefit. The psychiatric team can only keep him so long in the hospital, of course they're eager to hear anything he has to say regarding his ability to go back into the community. Where is the real help for the sick patients who think they're well because their illness tells them they are fine? The illness tells the patient that their loved ones are really the problem. The patients begin to hate and resent their loved ones for interfering, but how is the family supposed to keep themselves safe, and watch out for the safety of the community? None of this makes sense, and the family is left to pick up the pieces and put themselves back in harm's way.

So, with no help coming from his psychiatric team at home, I'm forced to drive Daniel back to our home once again. It's January, and I am thinking, "Do I put him out on the streets in the dead of winter, am I safe if we let him in our home?" We're no closer to finding help and we're no closer to stabilizing Daniel. It's just one Band-Aid after another placed on his psychic wounds in the hopes we might stumble on a moment or two of sanity in a day.

# CHAPTER FOUR:

## Keep My Son Far Away from Me

———◆———

*Tearless grief bleeds inwardly.*
*Christian Nestell Bovee*

Three days later on January 18, 2010, I receive my first death threat from Daniel. I find he's thrown out his medicine again because the voices are telling him he's well and we're trying to control him.

When I realize what he's done, I tell him, "We need to re-order your medications and I'll have to use your money to pay for them because you need to comply with your LRA, and dad and I don't have the money."

Daniel looks at me with contempt. "It makes me want to kill you. You don't think I'll do it, do you?"

Looking into his eyes, feeling his hatred, and with a chill running down my spine, I reply, "I know you want to, but then you'll end up in jail, not the mental hospital."

"Oh, you think so do you?" he says with a smirk on his face.

I'm stunned. I think Daniel knows he really isn't held to any sort of culpable responsibility in his life. He knows he can say anything to his medical team and they'll jump at his statements because they can only keep him for a limited time in a hospital bed…they need an out too. He knows he can work his way out of a murder conviction and he won't spend any time in jail. My blood runs cold as I look at my son I held so lovingly in my arms only 28 years earlier. My mind is swimming and I wonder, "Who is this person, and how can he really be threatening me with my life?" I decide I need my husband to intervene and I walk outside to phone Leonard and ask him to come home. This is the first time I've called Leonard at work and asked him to run interference.

When Leonard hears what's happened he says, "This is enough. I'll be right home." My husband determines we need to consider my safety. We go out that day with a mission to find Daniel an apartment and move him out of our home as quickly as possible.

I tell Leonard, "I am finally there. I'm ready to move him away. I feel like there's nothing more I can do to help Daniel."

We find an apartment on the second day of hunting; now we have to wait for the complex to finish the repairs being made to the unit before we move him in. We understand that we'll need to pay for most of the costs of his apartment, electricity, food, furniture, etc., because his supplemental security income won't cover much of the cost. I am thankful I'm still working, and my boss is understanding of this medical hardship. With my salary supplementing our family's income, we can afford to move Daniel into a new living space and out of our home.

At this point, I pray, "God keep my son as far away from me as possible." Daniel isn't trustworthy, he's full of horrible delusions and hallucinations and he truly frightens me. He's no longer in any reality that is apparent to a sane person. He paces outside, walking in circles around our kitchen island, talking and laughing with the invisible people. They talk to him and tell him what to think and feel. They're filling his mind with thoughts and making us the enemy, me in particular.

"I know that I should've walked away last year and left him on the street." I tell Leonard. Many people with mentally ill loved ones do just that. The struggle is too tough and the sick family member is too lost to reach any more. I hold my breath and count the days until we can move Daniel out. I am sleeping really lightly and awaken at the slightest noise. I pray I don't wake to find him standing over me. I find that I no longer care about his well-being. I'm worn out and done. No amount of effort on his behalf has come to any fruition. All my efforts are for nothing.

Leonard and I contact a friend and her husband and ask for their help in using their truck to move Daniel into his apartment. We move him in on January 30, 2010. He refuses to give us an apartment key and wants us gone. His hostility is palpable towards me and I am glad to get as far away from him as possible. As we drive off, I feel such guilt that I'm completely overwhelmed. I know this isn't in Daniel's best interest, but my fear overwhelms me with a need to get away from my child. I know in my heart that Daniel's psychosis will now overtake him because he won't have anyone near him to ground him in sanity. He'll be lost in his aloneness with the voices, hallucinations, and delusions. I fear for him and I fear for the community. This whole scenario is an extreme contrast to the sad farewell with Karis four months earlier. With Karis my heart is breaking for the lost time, talks, hugs, and memories I am missing out on. I fear for her safety because I don't know her roommates, the location of her home, or if it's safe in the house. These are all normal fears a mom has when her daughter walks out the door to go live in a location that is far away. With Daniel, I must confess, I worried about the location and the safety of his apartment, but also for the safety of the community. I feel great relief knowing I'll come home to a safe place where he is not. He's worn me down, and I have quit…I give up.

I called the psychiatric team and let them know, "We moved Daniel away from our home for my safety, after he threatened to kill me." They make a note of this in his chart, but there's no conversation about the situation. It's astonishing to me that he isn't brought in for care. It shocks me that they'll leave him in an apartment on his own. It's scary to know this sick person is left in the community untethered by loving hands.

I spend the next month rarely seeing Daniel, hoping his behavior towards me will improve as more time goes by. My husband is the main point of contact now, checking in on Daniel from time to time during each week. When Leonard gets home in the evenings after checking on Daniel he lets me know, "Each time I stop in the place is full of empty beer cans."

We both know that Daniel doesn't have money so we wonder how he's getting the beer, which of course is a violation of his LRA. Daniel's case manager checks on him in his apartment and makes sure he's taking his medication each day. We know she's seeing the tremendous amount of beer cans all through his place. I am stunned he hasn't been hospitalized due to the alcohol, the threat to kill me, and the breaking of his LRA. I ask my husband, "What will it take to push him into care again? Does someone in the community need to be hurt?"

I keep in touch with Karen and let her know what we're seeing with Daniel. She informs me that she checks on him and is helping him take his medication every day. She tells me, "Not everyone lives in a clean environment, and his apartment may not look like your home."

I wonder what that has to do with anything. I am not worried about the trash; I'm worried about the alcohol and how it is affecting Daniel's medication and his ability to think clearly through the voices. Luckily, his apartment is just one block from Grace Center so Karen can stop by easily, which is a major reason why we chose the location. I tell Karen everything that's happening, what my husband is seeing, and I explain to her our reasoning for moving Daniel out of our home.

Once a week, Leonard brings Daniel out to our house to visit. During one visit as I'm about to leave for the grocery store, Daniel asks, "Can I ride along?"

He seems stable during the visit, so after looking over at Leonard to get his read on the situation, I tell him, "Sure, you can come along."

While we're driving in the car, Daniel starts talking to me about being a porn star. He says, "I'm a porn star just like you were when you were in your twenties."

I look over at him confused, "I was never a porn star, but I did model in my teens and twenties." It's strange to hear him talk like that. He just puts his head back and starts laughing in a freaky sort of way.

In our attempt to keep Daniel eating, we buy him groceries and Leonard takes them by his apartment. He's losing a lot of weight, and you can tell he isn't eating much. My husband takes food over in the daytime when he thinks Daniel will be awake so he can talk to him and gauge how he's doing by his responses. For me, I go on my own to drop off cigarettes and food when I know he's asleep. I have a great fear of him because I know he believes the voices are real, they have his best interest in mind, and are giving him directions. His logic and rational thought are gone. In this setting I have no idea how he might act, or respond to anything. I do know the voices are trying to isolate him from me, and they're making me out as the problem. His days and nights are backwards and he normally wakes up around 3 PM or later. Daniel never locks his apartment door and many times I find it standing wide open with him asleep on his bed. If I see he's awake, I leave without him seeing me.

There are times when I have my husband take the groceries by the apartment because I assume Daniel may be awake. I don't want to be alone with him. He isolates me and then says stuff to me that he would never attempt to say if Leonard was around. As a mom, how is it that I can walk away from him when he's in such a psychotic state? How can I turn my back on my child in need? I struggle with these thoughts throughout my day.

The way I process it is to ask myself, "What will the trauma be to my family if Daniel commits a crime against me, possibly killing me?" The impact will be huge. I have other family members who need me in their lives. They would never forgive Daniel and the fracture would be irrevocable. The emotional pain would destroy the family.

I talk with Karis by phone almost every day. She calls me as she's walking home from her bus stop. It's a great time to catch up on her day, and know that all is well with her. Karis tells me she wants me to stay away from Daniel, she can't stand to think of me seeing him all alone. She goes on to say, "Daniel's threatening your life and he's incredibly sick. He's telling you what he's going to do to you. I work with people all day who live out this scenario and the worst case happens. If he hurts you, I may not be able to recover from it."

Each time she hears that I've gone to Daniel's apartment alone, she hangs up on me mid-sentence. At first it stuns me, then I realize it's her only way to communicate her frustration and fear. Karis still works in Minneapolis in restraining order court, and she's so far away that she's disconnected from our daily lives. She helps people apply for restraining orders, takes pictures of their injuries, and sits with them throughout the court proceedings. She hears horror stories of scenarios just like the one our family is going through. She's so afraid the same things may happen to our family. She knows if it were to happen, the family would not recover. I don't blame her, I understand. I explain to her that when she's a mom maybe she will understand why I can't turn away 100%. I worry about Daniel every day and wonder what hell he's living in at the moment.

Love is always a gift, but it can get dirty. I feel like I've walked this hard road for so long and I don't have any other source to tap for stamina. During this time, I feel such a disconnection from Daniel and I can't seem to reconnect. I never know what he's thinking or what he might say that will rock my world and put me into an adrenaline overload. I can feel my scalp tingle and my body get hot. I know it isn't healthy for me to feel the physical manifestations of fear and stress over the years. God has His part to do, and we need to do our part. We need to recognize our role. We need to be smart in how we put ourselves out there in the midst of mental illness. I constantly measure my thoughts and logic against how God wants us to care for our family and community. I know He doesn't want us to not put ourselves in potentially harmful situations. We can't just blindly walk forward into predicaments we should have considered before-hand. We need to be good stewards of our own safety. There's a time to cut losses and walk away to regroup our thoughts and motives.

My husband brings Daniel out to the house one weekend. I've just come home from visiting Karis in Minneapolis for four days and I am looking forward to seeing Daniel and checking on his well-being. Leonard is becoming more alarmed at Daniel's state of uncleanliness, his appearance, and the volume of beer cans taking over his apartment each time Leonard arrives to pick him up for an outing. We have a nice visit at our home and he seems to be in a pretty good place. He's walking in pain with every step, and grimacing. He's bent over in pain and looks like he's 90 years old.

He says, "It's growing pains causing me to hurt."

We can see his health is clearly deteriorating and I ask him, "Are you eating?"

I wonder if the pain is from malnourishment. He remains in pain, and is hobbling the entire day he's with us. I'm told he's been this way for at least one to two weeks. This lets me know his caregivers have to see this when they come by to administer his medications.

Daniel asks me, "Will you drive me home?"

After looking at Leonard to see his expression and if he thinks it safe, I agree. I figure Daniel's been great today with us and it'll be okay. I tell my husband, "I'll take Daniel by the store and get him some vitamins and then drop him at his apartment."

We pull into Right Drugs to grab him some supplements that I'm hoping he'll take to help him with his nutrition levels. As we're walking through the drug store, I let Daniel know, "I hope you're feeling better soon...I think these vitamins may help with the pain." And finally I ask him, "Do you think you should try and eat more?" He's getting so thin, he now weighs about 135 pounds and he's 5 feet 11 inches tall. We purchase the vitamins and head outside and get back in the car.

I tell him, "I'm sorry you're in such pain. I wish I could take it away."

I look over at him while I am pulling out of the parking lot, and he tells me, "You are one hot fuck."

I feel sick to my stomach and look over at Daniel. He's leaning against the front seat passenger car door with his body fully turned to look at me head on with an evil, lustful look on his face. By this time, I'm driving past the front of a grocery store and I feel my heart literally skip beats. My mind goes blank. All I can say is, "Oh, Daniel."

In my stunned state, I think to myself, should I pull over into the grocery store parking lot and make him get out, or should I go the last few miles in silence and drop him at his apartment? It's early February and very cold. I think, "If I just keep looking forward out the front windshield, and don't respond to him, I just may make it to a place where I can drop him off safely." As I keep driving I ask myself, "Can I hurt him if he tries anything? What will I do? How will I do it? Do I think I'm strong enough?" All of these thoughts are roiling through my mind. I am praying silently for God's protection while I finish the last few blocks. I can't bring myself to look at Daniel again and I don't say a word. I can see from my peripheral vision he's silently sitting there, leaning against the door leering at me, and smiling. He hasn't moved or said another thing since he made the statement and the look on his face is devastating to me.

I pull up in front of his apartment and just sit there without looking at him. No words have passed between us. He takes the bag of vitamins and gets out of the car and shuts the door. I immediately put the car in drive and get out of there. I start shaking and crying after I get out of the apartment complex and away from him. I pull the car over in the parking lot of a burger joint and cry. This is a person I don't know, and I don't want to know. Is this who we're going to end up with after Dr. Egan integrates all the voices in Daniel's head into one persona? I am in big trouble and so is the community.

I go back to Daniel's apartment really early the next morning on my way to work because he left his cigarettes at our home the evening before, and I know he'll need them. I am going to hang them on the doorknob and get out of there as fast as I can because Leonard is now out of town. I find his door wide open, and he's awake. He says hello with a normal smile on his face and seems very warm and caring. I go in and I'm shocked at the state of the apartment. This is the first time I've been in his apartment since moving day, and it's filthy and filled with trash. Leaving the door wide open, I start cleaning out the garbage and end up with nine large thirty-gallon trash bags of mostly beer cans. While I'm cleaning his unit, I find some paperwork from the County Court House showing he was arrested for stealing beer from Right Drugs.

I ask Daniel about the documents and he tells me, "I went into Right Drugs drunk one afternoon and stole a case of beer. I walked out to the grassy area in front of the store and sat down with the unopened beer, and passed out. The police were called and I was arrested and taken to the court house and was booked into jail."

I find out later that after he was booked and in the holding cell, they recognized him as mentally ill and they phoned the Grace Center and asked them to come get him. A case manager from Grace Center went in the next day and picked him up. I can see from the paperwork I'm holding that he was appointed an attorney to represent him. The lawyer is identified as being assigned to him from the Indigent Defense Panel for District Court Defendants. Her name is Ms. Ellen Ridgley. Ms. Ridgley becomes a huge legal support to our family in the process and outcome of the legal charges against Daniel.

I am stunned the case manager didn't take him to the Grace Center hospital for care, as he obviously broke his LRA again. My husband and I weren't notified about the arrest even though Daniel's psychiatric team knows we're his primary support system. If I had not potentially put myself in danger and gone into Daniel's apartment to bring him his cigarettes, I wouldn't have known this episode occurred.

As soon as I leave Daniel's apartment I call my husband to let him know what I found. We are sad once more to see his spiral into mental illness speeding up to a grave level. I leave Daniel's apartment with the arrest papers outlining the charges so I can show Leonard when he returns home from business travel. It's strange to see Daniel so completely detached from reality and not caring at all about anything.

When Leonard and I are finally able to talk to Daniel together, he's nonchalant and doesn't care about any impact to his life regarding the fact that he's starting down the road to a criminal record. He doesn't see any problem with the way his life is heading and he has no intention of being sober. He also believes he spent three to four days in jail. In fact, he only spent one night. It seems like all the hard work we put into trying to keep Daniel out of the legal system is failing. He can't see the long term problems coming from his behavior, and apparently his psychiatric team isn't worried or interested.

My coworker and friend, Jody, calls Daniel's case manager at Grace Center one morning the following week to see if they know that he was arrested for being drunk and stealing beer the week before. The case manager assures Jody, "Yes, we know and we're on it." Jody is quite shocked the LRA has no weight and Daniel's breaking the agreement has no ramifications. She can't believe

Daniel is still in the community and so gravely ill. She's also surprised at the lack of help we're receiving and she's growing frustrated right along with us. Jody used to work in the juvenile justice system in years past and is very helpful to have on this journey. She teaches me how to go online to look up the arrest information on Daniel and how to read and understand the charges. Her help is invaluable as we've never dealt with illegal activity or arrests before in our lives. I keep my eye on the records and court appointed dates for his hearing. I talk to Daniel about the charges and court dates but he isn't worried and doesn't cares about anything concerning the arrest.

It's at this time that I begin to think about how to get Daniel's rights revoked and get him legally under our care. Jody takes me to visit a judge and we discuss finding a lawyer who can help with this process, if we decide to go that route. The rate at which Daniel's decompensating is quite alarming. Nothing has worked so far and I'm beginning to lose all hope.

A couple days later during another visit to Daniel's apartment he tells me, "I hear the dead bodies in the cemetery next-door. They're knocking on the coffins trying to get out. Is there anything we can do to help them?"

I just look at him without a response. He's so sure about the hallucinations that reasoning with him makes him angry because the delusion is so much stronger than any reality. There's no reasoning or explaining the delusion away, so I stay silent.

After a few minutes, Daniel continues from out of nowhere, "I want to rape, sexually torture, murder, and then dismember your body."

I find myself shutting down and going non-responsive. I don't even know how I'm supposed to respond. Standing there it hits me that I am the one person his voices are fixated on destroying. I learned during the last sixteen years of hospital visits that the voices work to isolate and condemn the ill person to a lonely life where they lose their loved ones in a web of imagination and fantasy. If the voices can get me to leave and abandon Daniel, they'll win and have Daniel to themselves. The fantasy dreams will overwhelm what tenuous grasp of reality he still holds on to. While I am scared out of my wits, I know this isn't my son and I can't abandon him to the call of their voices; I'm not going to let them win. A mother's love for her child is an unrivaled force of nature.

Later that evening while I'm resting at home, I realize the knocking Daniel is hearing is probably coming from the residents all around him as he's probably listening to TV or music at a really loud level and yelling conversations with his voices. They are undoubtedly trying to get his attention to turn down the volume and quit screaming so they can sleep. Since he has his days and nights backward, the other residents are probably not getting any sleep and are becoming more frustrated and frightened of him each day.

As I see Daniel's grip on reality leaving him, I'm amazed his psychiatric team is making no efforts to step in and get him help. They can see the LRA is not upheld in so many ways, and from so many different angles. Karis encourages me, "Start a log of every event, every cry for help, all of your attempts at an intervention and requests for a bed, and mark down the outcomes of each, who you spoke to, along with the date and time. Keep it to protect our family in case Daniel ever harms anyone because then we can show our attempts to get help and the walls put up to prevent his care."

In this situation, so many times the community turns on the family, casting blame that they didn't prevent the tragedy. They want to know what the family did, or tried to do for help. If the worst happens and somebody is injured, I can produce my log with the 'who, what, when, where, and why' of the situation. The log will put the mental health community on the line for an explanation of their system and their processes. It will showcase the lack of support options we have in our community. We can't reverse the harm, but maybe it can bring about change for other mentally ill people and their families.

One afternoon in early March, Tyler calls me from work and asks me if I can bring some jumper cables out to his office and help jump his car. I let him know I'm on my way and I head out. As I leave work and start driving up Southwest Broadway, I see Daniel wandering down the sidewalk outside of Right Drug looking completely out of it. I am shocked to see him looking so bad. He's stumbling on the sidewalk, stooped over looking for cigarette butts on the ground. I keep on driving because I know I'm not supposed to be alone with him and he's really becoming more lost in his psychosis. I am afraid to be near him after the last week of strange behavior. As I drive further up the street I realize as a mother I can't leave him alone and insane on the sidewalk. If I don't look out for him, who will? I turn the car around in the Safeway parking lot at the end of the next block and I head back to pick him up.

However, when I get back to Right Drugs, Daniel is gone. My heart sinks because I know he can't get far as slowly as he's walking and it looks like each step still causes him so much pain. I immediately wonder if he's inside stealing beer again. As I look over towards the hotel next door, I see him hunting for used cigarette butts outside the hotel entrance. I pull up beside him and roll down my window and ask him, "Do you want a ride?"

When he gets in the car, he says, "Did they call you?"

With a perplexed look on my face I tell him, "I don't know what you're talking about."

"Never mind," he says and starts to laugh. His mind is fractured and he's incoherent. I let him know I'm going to see Tyler at his work and he's welcome to come with me. I figure it's only a couple miles up the road to Tyler and I will be just fine for the short distance.

Daniel's totally lost in his delusion. He's filthy, smells horrible, and his eyes look glassy and strange. In the car he tells me, "I tried to steal beer again today but they caught me. I gave it back and they let me leave. I've stolen beer five or six times. When they catch me stealing I give it back, and if they don't catch me then I have beer."

He goes on, "I assume Right Drugs called your cell to tell you I just tried to steal again today."

"Right Drugs doesn't have my cell phone number, and they don't know my name. They have no way to call me." I say.

He shifts the topic quickly, "I'm with the Mexican Mafia and I use cocaine. What can Right Drugs do about my stealing, considering my connections with the mafia?" He starts talking to the voices and throwing his head back and laughing out loud. He goes on and on about the mafia cocaine scenario and is totally convinced about this delusion. I am creeped out.

We arrive shortly at Tyler's work and I go in to the building with Daniel. It is a library for a University and Tyler's office is on an upper floor. I figure Daniel may pass for a student and no one will know he belongs with Tyler.

I ask Daniel, "Can I buy you some food out of the vending machine?" I can tell he hasn't eaten. He's so skinny and getting more emaciated every time I see him; his jeans are falling off of his hips. Daniel has me get him some chips and then scarfs them down and wants more. I am more than happy to keep buying the chips because I know it is at least some calories high in fat. When Tyler sees that Daniel is there, he suggests that we wait out by the car for AAA because he's appalled at the state Daniel is in.

We walk out to the broken-down Jeep and Daniel climbs in to wait for the tow truck. Tyler and I move over to my car to discuss the condition Daniel's in and what we should do with him. Tyler determines he'll drive Daniel back to his apartment and leave me with the Jeep to wait for AAA. We finish talking and approach the Jeep to let Daniel know our plans. Tyler gets in the car with Daniel and shuts the door. Such a look of revulsion takes over Tyler's face as he sees what Daniel has done, the smells coming off of him, and the fact that he has stripped out of his clothes and is talking incoherently with his voices and laughing. Daniel's totally lost to us at this point and we're at a loss because his psychiatric team has turned a blind eye to the arrest for stealing, drunkenness, physical emaciation, and incoherency. At this point, we've no options but to take him back to his apartment.

Tyler knows he has to be the one to take Daniel back to his apartment and get him away from me and away from his workplace. Tyler tells him, "Put your clothes back on," and he gets out of the car as fast as he can. Tyler looks stricken beyond words. He decides to take Daniel home, and stop by a drive through and buy him some food before he drops him off at his apartment.

"I'll take care of the Jeep and have dad come pick me up at the auto shop." I tell him.

I think this is the first time Tyler has seen the extent of Daniel's mental illness and he's shocked at the profound decline in his big brother. For their safety, Tyler keeps his family isolated from our home dynamics and Daniel's mental illness. This isn't the brother he knew from his childhood. They are only eighteen months apart in age and have such good memories of their childhood. Those memories are dashed this day. Tyler goes into protective mode for me and our families.

Tyler tells me this is the last straw. "I no longer want Daniel around my family unless I'm present. Either you or I have to be with my family if Daniel's around." Daniel is now a person Tyler no longer recognizes. Tyler heads out with Daniel and I take care of the car issues. It's a sober end to a normal work day. I know this type of thing happens to so many people who are also dealing with mental illness in their families. I wish it wasn't the norm, but unfortunately it is.

During the months of January and February, I read a book called Sociopath Next Door by Martha Stout, Ph.D., to see if Daniel has the tendencies of a sociopath. I am not sure because of his behavior and his ability to manipulate if a personality disorder is also at play along with his mental illness. By the end of book, I determine Daniel isn't a sociopath. When you're caught in this situation it's so hard to know if you are being manipulated while you're also being traumatized. Reading the book helps me know Daniel doesn't show the traits of a sociopath. I'm able to lay this fear to rest and concentrate on his mental illness and finding help from that view point.

I'm at a point of profound alienation from my faith. Do I walk away from God? I don't understand the lack of healing for Daniel. I feel abandoned and ignored in my prayers. I don't get why he isn't made whole to live out a life that will bring him peace, where he can make an impact. I've taken to thinking of Daniel as dead, otherwise I can't keep functioning. It's easier to let things go when you think the person no longer exists. It takes tremendous willpower to think of him as dead. Many tears were shed for such a beautiful soul lost to me. Now what are my options, walk away from my faith which has helped me every step of the way since I was 14 years old, just because my life isn't unfolding how I envisioned? What do I walk to? There's nothing the world has that I want; it is lost in self-absorption and false ideology. It holds no place for me and won't meet the spiritual needs I have as a human being.

After years of soul searching and railing against God, I realize I must decide to change my perspective. I know I have to look at things differently and ask God to use me as a tool of learning and open my mind up to absorb the knowledge of my unending research to help recover our son. I know the mental health system isn't going to do it for me. I can't even get Daniel's psychiatric team to make positive moves when an obvious breach of his least restrictive alternative agreement is made. I know it's going to take a major traumatic event to get his psychiatric team to open their eyes and move forward in a way that will bring Daniel relief. I change my prayers to, "God teach me, lead me, and enlighten my thinking. Show me what I need to know and help me pull the string and unravel Your truths. Open my mind to understand. Whatever You want to do with me, I will trust." I have to root down and have these ugly honest talks with God in prayer.

On March 10, 2010, the Colonial Apartments where Daniel lives calls my husband at noon. Brad, the manager for the apartment complex leaves a message asking him to call back. Leonard phones Brad and immediately leaves work to go to Daniel's apartment complex after hearing that Daniel is nude outside his apartment.

Brad tells my husband that he instructed Daniel, "Get your clothes on, you can't be outside nude." He walked away from

Daniel and immediately called my husband. The apartment complex has Leonard sign a form saying if Daniel's behavior doesn't change in the next three days, he'll be evicted. When my husband gets to Daniel's private apartment, he finds him oblivious to any wrongdoing.

"Are you going to change how you're acting?" Leonard asks Daniel incredulously. "You can't be nude outside the apartment… it's illegal. You'll be thrown in jail, or out on the streets, if you don't comply with the apartment complex's request for you to follow their rules."

Daniel's only response is, "Whatever happens, happens."

The ramifications of the situation escape Daniel. My husband calls me after he finished talking with the apartment manager and Daniel. He's amazed Daniel has no worries about anything. Our son is truly in his own world and doesn't care what anyone does to him.

This same afternoon I put together a teleconference with my husband and Karen Everett. Leonard and I phone Karen from our different offices so we can discuss the path forward with Daniel because his behavior is becoming more erratic and bizarre, not to mention illegal.

Once I got the three of us connected I kick off the conversation, "Daniel's getting worse by the day. We haven't experienced illegal behavior until now, and I believe Daniel is really under medicated. Can we get a medication change for Daniel, because being on only 2mg of Abilify isn't cutting it? He's overwhelmed by voices, delusions and hallucinations, and we can't get through to him." I continue after taking a quick breath, "We're lucky Daniel wasn't arrested for lewd conduct for sunbathing nude outside his apartment door, believing he's a porn star." I can feel my heart rate sky rocketing and I feel so helpless in the face of these changes.

Karen calmly replies, "I'm not a doctor so I can't speak to the under medication statement you just made."

"I'm not a doctor either but I know a gravely mentally ill patient when I see one, and Daniel is severely ill and he's not medicated correctly." I respond emphatically.

"Diane," Leonard interjects, "you need to calm down because Karen isn't the enemy."

I didn't realize my voice had risen so high and I work to pull back my anger and try and remain rational and logical so we can get something positive happening for Daniel.

Karen goes on, "I'll work on a remedy to the out of control situation and discuss Daniel's medication with the doctor. The previous week I saw Daniel outside his apartment nude when I stopped by to give him his medications. I asked him to put his clothes on and told him it wasn't okay to be outside naked."

I can hardly contain myself when I hear that she saw him nude outside his apartment and didn't say anything or do anything for his safety. My response is swift and heated, "How can you see a mentally ill person outside sunbathing in the nude and just ask him to put his clothes on and make no effort to intervene on his behalf?! You saw him breaking the law and just walked away!"

I hear Leonard on his end of the conference call again trying to calm me down, telling me, "Karen is on our side; she can help us resolve this crisis."

I feel alone and lost in a fragmented system. My mind is spinning with so many thoughts. Bottom line: Daniel is as much a victim as the community. In this type of situation, Daniel is just as likely to be victimized as he is to victimize someone; in his illness he would welcome the abuse. This is a lose/lose situation and I'm at a loss for how to turn this around. The system which is built as an advocacy for the mentally ill isn't functioning as it should, and the mentally ill have no champion for their well-being within the state and federal system. The family is left holding everything together in the hopes they can keep their family members and the community safe from any harm.

Karen lets us know she will talk with the doctor and get back with us. I feel a grief so severe that I feel I won't make it through the day. How can Daniel have spiraled down so low that he's naked outside his apartment, believes he's filming a porn movie, and finds no problem with his behavior? We bring Daniel out to our home to stay in the evening because we know he can't stay in the community like he is because he could end up nude outside his apartment again. As much as I fear him, I also fear for his safety. He's still my child and there's nowhere for us to turn to for help. Everything within the system failed us and we're the only ones to house Daniel and pray for a breakthrough.

CHAPTER FIVE:

# The Beginning

———◆———

*A blessed thing it is for any man or woman to have a friend, one human soul whom we can trust utterly, who knows the best and worst of us, and who loves us in spite of all our faults.*
*Charles Kingsley*

As I find myself standing on the precipice of the unknown, I need to stop myself and remember to look back to the good times. The times when our lives seemed full of promise each day; and there was no psychological pain, a time when our lives seemed easy and my life wasn't threatened by my son. Back to a time before I found myself thinking, "If I can just get to work where we have security guards and metal detectors then I'll feel safe because my son can't reach me." Back to a time when I didn't need to wait to go home until my husband was also set to arrive because I was afraid of being alone with my son.

I want to go back to a world that was ours for the choosing. I want to look upon my son with hope and happiness each morning. I want to return to a time when there is still potential and he can help sway his future by his own decisions, a time when Daniel has a chance at sanity and his mind doesn't fail him when he needs it most. To survive, I hold on to the ever present fact that great love flourishes in our home.

# CHAPTER SIX:

## Keep My Son Forever in Our Arms

———◆———

*Know that wisdom is such to your soul; if you find it, there will be a future,*
*and your hope will not be cut off.*
*Proverbs 24:14*

It's June 1981. My husband and I have been married two years and we're expecting our first child. These are the days when parents don't get to know the sex of their baby before the birth; it doesn't matter and it's not an option anyway. The surprise comes instantly at birth when they announce, "it's a boy," or "it's a girl."

I wake Leonard up in the early hours of the morning telling him, "I am bleeding more than normal." I'm only thirty-eight weeks pregnant but the baby is coming soon. I was told earlier in my pregnancy that the placenta was attached very low in my uterus and was partially obstructing the cervix. There's a chance that as the baby grows, it will cause the placenta to stretch and move enough to allow the cervix to dilate and offer me the opportunity to have a natural childbirth. While we wait for the months to pass, I have moments where I bleed almost monthly, and worry I won't be able to carry our child to a healthy delivery. Leonard and I are very excited for our first baby and we wait in anticipation for the birth. We attend Lamaze childbirth classes and learn breathing and relaxation techniques in expectation of the big moment. My husband and I grab my pre-packed suitcase and my special focal point that I picked which will enable me to concentrate while performing Lamaze breathing techniques. My focal point is a picture of Leonard and me, smiling and in love. We're both so young and excited for the new journey of our marriage. We dated for six years before marrying and now we're heading to the hospital to welcome our first family member.

Upon arrival, the doctor checks me and says, "You'll need to remain in the hospital and stay in bed in the hopes the bleeding stops." Unfortunately, by 6 PM that evening with the bleeding continuing, the doctor decides for the safety of the baby, they'll need to break my water and get the birth going. We feel prepared and ready for a natural childbirth. We're ready to put the breathing techniques to work and get this done.

The contractions start quickly after the doctor breaks my water. It takes all my concentration and my husband's coaching efforts to keep me going. I don't want any pain medication and epidurals for childbirth don't exist at this time. I know pain medication will cause our baby to become sedated at birth and I want an alert baby, ready to breathe and meet us for the first time. There aren't any monitors or probes placed on the baby's skull or around my abdomen as I labor. It is all peaceful and calm.

As I enter transition (7–10cm), I can't believe how intense the pain is. I'm having trouble keeping up with the breathing and enduring the pain. I start to hyperventilate and need to breathe into a paper bag to bring my $CO_2$ levels back to normal. It works and I find myself going internal to deal with the whole thing, praying for it to be over.

Finally, four hours of total labor later, the nurse checks me and says, "You can start pushing, you're ten centimeters." The baby is birthed within fifteen minutes. It's a miracle to hear the doctor say, "It's a boy."

Those four hours are the most painful hours of my life, but I now hold a beautiful baby boy. The pain is worth the gift. Holding my baby and looking into his face is such a peaceful moment. I'm the first person to hug and hold my son, and he steals my heart.

My husband and I name our beautiful baby boy, Daniel Clay Jackson Borders. We tried to conceive for two years and didn't know if we'd be able to have other children, so we gave him all the names we liked. We're so blessed and we're flying high. God performed a miracle and we have our son.

The hospital keeps Daniel in the nursery because moms aren't allowed to have their babies in their rooms with them in the early 1980s. I only receive him for nursing periodically throughout the day, so I walk to the nursery and stand at the window and tell anyone and everyone who walks by that I have the most beautiful baby boy in the whole world. I'm smitten. He's precious and vulnerable; we'll protect and raise him in a home full of love and promise. The world is his for the taking, and Leonard and I will work to bring possibilities his way.

Daniel grows up to be a quiet, kind, and gentle young child. He's introverted and shy and has a few close friends. I teach him to read early on and he reads on his own constantly. His favorite book is Wake Up Sun by David L. Harrison. While he's in his elementary school years, I attend night college classes taking chemistry and mathematics. He sits by my side while I use flash cards to memorize the periodic table of elements and their charges. He ends up memorizing them right along with me. Even now, twenty-five years in the future, he retains this knowledge of the periodic table. He's a brilliant young child and absorbs everything around him. Throughout his younger years, Daniel makes such an impact on his cousin Melanie that she names her first child, a baby girl, Sydney Dani.

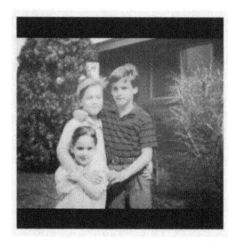

Daniel often says he wants to attend the Massachusetts Institute of Technology and learn mathematics, chemistry, and physics. In the eighth grade he goes to a summer camp class at the local community college to continue learning math at a faster pace than what's being taught in the public school system. He's gifted in the sciences and we encourage his dreams.

As a way to boost his self-esteem and get him out into the world and around potential new friends, we use one of Leonard's work bonuses to pay for martial arts classes for Daniel. He starts martial arts at the age of nine and continues until age fifteen. He's quick and strong and he's very proud of himself. The classes really boost his self-esteem. His younger brother Tyler and his sister Karis are proud to have Daniel as a sibling. No one wants to mess with Tyler or Karis because they know how tough Daniel is in martial arts. He holds the U.S. Championship record for breaking four one-inch boards with one kick while he was still in grade school. He rises to a level within martial arts where he's teaching three to four times a week, and also attending classes. Our family takes Daniel on a trip to Albany, Oregon, for a martial arts competition. He wins many awards and trophies for this one-day competition. As the years roll by, he completes his first degree black belt and is just one test away from his second degree black belt when he begins not wanting to attend classes or teach.

His kindness and compassion is an everyday constant, but his shyness and quietness keeps him from being part of a bigger crowd. Childhood can be cruel. It's hard for a parent to watch the effects of peer pressure, the choosing of sides, and the deliberate hurt that children inflict on each other. It's hard to know when to step in and when to let a learning experience happen. Where is the line drawn to protect your child? We know something is wrong. His demeanor is changing; we're losing him and don't know why.

In April of 1995, out of nowhere it seems like a light switch is thrown and the Daniel I know is gone. No longer do I see my son in his eyes but a stranger with no compassion, dead and dark. My husband is working in Boston when the change happens, a nondescript day in April. I remember sensing something was different but not believing it with my mind. How can a child change so fast? Did something happen at school that I should know about? He begins wearing only black clothing. I find him with his fingernails painted black and black liner around his eyes. He's so angry and difficult to reach.

He comes to me one day and asks, "Can I have ten dollars to buy a jacket from a kid at school." He says he really likes the jacket and it's a great deal, so I give him the money. To my surprise he walks in the door that afternoon when school gets out and is wearing a green German field jacket. He begins styling his hair slicked back and becomes obsessed with anything to do with Adolph Hitler. He spends a lot of time reading about World War II and Stalin. He quotes facts of World War II from both sides of the war and knows statistics that I'm amazed he's learned.

Daniel also starts to take on the family history and life struggles of Nirvana's Kurt Cobain. Cobain is central in the punk and grunge scene in Seattle, Washington, and Daniel can't get enough of him. He begins imagining the same family offenses and issues against our family that he reads about Kurt's family. He sits in his room for hours listening to Cobain's album Nevermind and the hit single "Smells Like Teen Spirit" over and over and over. Daniel tells me, "I won't live past the age of 30; I will die young." He listens to the anti-establishment rants of Kurt Cobain and gets lost in that world.

It's in this timeframe when Tyler grabs me one evening and asks me, "Will you look through Daniel's room? There are notes you need to find." I never dig through the rooms of our three children because I trust them and we share great relationships. We talk often and they know they don't need to hide anything; I love them unconditionally. However, that evening when Daniel leaves to teach martial arts, I go into his room and start looking through his drawers and under his bed. I find notes where he's talking about suicide and he has homicidal ideations towards his brother. I'm stunned! What caused Daniel's mind to warp so quickly? I don't know this Daniel, and I am at a loss as to what I should do.

I contact my work insurance and they put me in touch with the Employee Assistance Program that specializes in working issues like this one. The next morning, I have an appointment to bring Daniel to meet with Woody, a counselor suggested by the program. This is our first mental health meeting and I have no idea what I am going to be facing in the future. I have no knowledge of what mental illness even is, let alone how to find help. I don't think we have a family history of mental illness so I'm clueless.

Daniel talks with Woody a few times and he comes to the conclusion that Daniel is suffering from major depression. He recommends that I take Daniel to a psychiatrist for further care. I remember walking out of these appointments with Woody wondering what's happening. I am out of my sphere of comfort, and I have no idea what's going on. I have no frame of reference of which to lay this experience.

When I call my mother and father to discuss what's taking place with Daniel, I find out I do have schizophrenia on both my mom and dad's side of the family. My mom's aunt tried to drown her baby girl in the bathtub and was committed to a psychiatric hospital for a time. After she was released, she was found again trying to drown her baby. My great aunt will live out the remainder of her years in a psychiatric hospital in Oregon and eventually die in the same hospital. My father's side of the family has schizophrenia plaguing its offspring too. My cousin's son has schizophrenia and he's about five years older than Daniel. It's truly amazing how well families hide mental illness as if it's a shame, a character flaw. This is the 1990s and nobody talks about this sort of thing, except to blame the families of the ill (mostly the mom), or to claim it's the work of the Devil.

In early fall of 1995, Daniel tries to convince Karis the stories he's made up in his mind are actually true and he wants to impress them on Karis and skew her perception of reality. I'm furious when I find Daniel working on her psychologically in the van when I go in to the middle school to pick up Tyler from basketball practice. As I get into the van and see Karis's expression, I ask her, "Are you okay?"

She looks scared and confused and begins to tell me, "Daniel says you're hurting him, and me too… all of us."

When I hear what he's said, I turn to Daniel and tell him, "If I ever catch you doing or saying anything like this again, no matter how much I love you, I will force you out of our home because I won't have you telling your stories to your little sister. She has no ability to process the lies you're telling and make sense of them."

This situation is really hard on me because Karis adores her brother and they're close. She's too young to understand the changes coming over Daniel and his manipulation is very confusing to her. She has no ability to handle a teenage brother who's always been well before and now tells stories which don't make sense. I realize this is a very tenuous position to be in and I wonder what he's saying to other people in general, and if he's convincing them too that he's in the same kind of household as Kurt Cobain.

Daniel begins carving words in the flesh on his arms, and one evening I walk into his room to find him sitting on his bed and inserting needles underneath his fingernails. I guess in some people with mental issues this is a common practice. His new psychiatrist calls it cutting. Daniel has a vacant look on his face and seems lost and alone. I sit with him and try to let him know how much we love him and are here for him.

I prompt him, "Let's talk about anything you want, we can discuss anything you're upset about."

He looks at me in an empty way and doesn't respond. He's far away and his eyes aren't focusing on anything. This is so far removed from the relationship we've always shared. He and I have always been so close. We both love to read books and discuss science and talk about everything. He's brilliant and gifted, and can learn anything. Now, he's pushing me away and placing walls up so I can't reach him. He's such a handsome young man and he has the world at his feet. I'm starting to see a shell of a person with no life. This is so far out of my understanding and I don't have any frame of reference with which to compare this. I'm lost and afraid and am hoping the psychiatrist can help Daniel and bring him back to where he was prior to this switch. I pray for God to please keep my son safe from whatever is plaguing his mind.

Daniel and I meet with his new psychiatrist, Dr. Douglas Donovan, in the fall of 1995. I spend fifteen minutes with Daniel and the doctor and then he asks me to step out of the room for the next thirty-five minutes. Dr. Donovan brings me back in at the end of the appointment to regroup and talk about the path forward. He says he'll need to see Daniel frequently and we get him set up for weekly visits. Daniel also starts on psychiatric medication to help with his depression and suicidal thinking.

While we wait for the next weekly appointment, I find Daniel in his room loading and unloading a shotgun to practice his speed. He's timing himself to get faster. He's sitting in front of his bedroom window with the curtains up so he has the light shining down on him and when I walk in it's like he's bathed in sunshine. I don't even know where my husband stores the guns let alone know that Daniel has a weapon. My blood runs cold and I catch my breath and process what my mind is seeing.

I approach him slowly and calmly ask, "What are you doing sweetie?"

His response comes slowly after a long pause. Then he says, "I need to get faster at loading the gun." His voice is without inflexion and is very distant.

"Can I please have the gun? It's really dangerous and I want you safe." I gently ask him. As I walk out of his bedroom with the gun, I know I have to get all the weapons out of our home. I wonder about knives too. Do I need to clear the house of knives, baseball bats? After all, it's not the object that kills, it's the person behind the weapon and their state of mind, and their delusional thinking that does the killing. Will I awake in the night to find him hurting our family? Are we in immediate danger? I know I'm in way over my head and the psychiatrist is my lifeline.

I am grateful for the second visit with Dr. Donovan and am very hopeful for good results. I know I need to share with him what happened between visits. I sit in the waiting room hoping the doctor will call me in at the end of the appointment to talk with me and see how I feel Daniel is doing. Eventually, the doctor comes out and asks me to come back into his office with Daniel. Much to my surprise, I learn Daniel has woven stories to this doctor just as he tried to do with Karis. Unfortunately, he believes the stories at face value. He hasn't met my husband or our other children and only talked with me for fifteen minutes the week before, so how can he make this call?

Dr. Donovan tells me in a stoic, cold manner, "You and your husband are the cause of Daniel's mental illness. He's suffering from Post-Traumatic Stress Disorder. Your parenting is the issue."

He calmly continues to unravel my world, "I don't want you to drive Daniel to these appointments. He can take the bus."

My response is quick, "There's no way Daniel will be riding the bus, it's winter and snowing. The bus route is a two-hour trip, and I can drive him in fifteen minutes on the back roads from our home."

"Daniel is self-medicating with cigarettes and you need to buy them and give him some to help him stay calm every day. He'll be subject to random urine tests for hard narcotics and if any are found in his system, I'll pull Daniel from your home and place him in foster care because you are the problem."

The doctor knows Daniel is smoking marijuana and that is fine with him because again Daniel is just self-medicating. I'm stunned to hear the doctor tell me I need to allow Daniel to break two laws, allow smoking and purchase the cigarettes for him, and turn a blind eye to marijuana, but he better not graduate to any harder drugs or he is to be stripped from our home and his care taken over by the state. What in the world is going on? I feel like Alice in Wonderland. I walk out of this appointment in a daze. Truthfully, I can't even think. I feel a cold chill run down my spine when I realize the damage that can happen to our home and to our children by an out of control system. Being a newbie to the mental health system, I am at a total loss of what to do to repair this situation. I have nowhere to turn, and no one to talk to. A few people I know suggest "Just put Daniel into foster care and change your locks to keep the family safe from the trauma of the situation he's promoting."

I drive back to work after I drop Daniel at home following the appointment. I am not processing well, I'm still in a state of shock. I have no memory of leaving the doctor's office or how I got Daniel home. I call my father from the parking lot at work when I arrive and proceed to tell him about what just happened at the psychiatrist office.

I blurt out, "Leonard and I are to blame for Daniel's mental illness." I'm crying and explaining what I was told. When you're forced to look at yourself as the cause of such psychiatric pain in your loved one you find yourself numb. This is the doctor that knows it all, he's the psychiatrist. I am just a mom doing her best to raise her children correctly and with love.

I ask my dad, "What did I do that was so harmful? I wasn't told anything specific, just that we caused the damage." I remember back to Daniel weaving fantasy delusions about our home life to Karis, and I realize he's doing the same thing with the psychiatrist who is buying all of it without proof or follow-up. I thank God my wonderful, loving dad talk's sense back into me.

Dad tells me, "You and Leonard are great parents and only ever had Daniel's best interest at heart." It helps ground me back into knowing that Leonard and I are okay, and Daniel is just sick.

My dad goes on, "You stayed home after his birth and were home for fourteen years raising your babies in the most secure environment, full of love and support. You and Leonard are not the problem. The guy is a quack."

Hearing his affirming words anchor me back to earth and my heart feels like it might beat normally again. I find it inexcusable this doctor can level such charges and such threats in the face of no proof. When I was confronted with the stark words of the doctor, my mind just shut down. I realize the doctor has an agenda, and it's not in the interest of our family ending intact. I also know any overt move on my part to remove Daniel from his care will result in him initiating the state to come into our home and remove him from our care. I am in a no win situation and my options are nonexistent. The psychiatrist holds all the power, and the state is at his call whenever the hard drugs show up in Daniel's system. This situation can implode so quickly with Daniel hanging with people selling drugs and willing to sell him anything he asks for. How is this going to play out if he decides to try something harder?

The next few weeks pass in a fog for me. I have no idea what Daniel's saying to the doctor because I'm not allowed in during the hour long doctor's visit. I sit outside in the car with the engine idling trying to keep warm with snow all around, waiting for Daniel to come out of his sessions. The doctor never asks for me and doesn't want to hear what I see or experience with my son. Daniel somehow continues to use marijuana and it shows up in his urine tests, but the doctor pays it no mind. He really is fine with my fourteen-year-old getting high on marijuana and smoking cigarettes.

One day following a visit with Dr. Donovan, Daniel comes out to the car and says, "The doctor told me I'll never have a relationship with dad and reconciliation isn't possible."

What in the world is Daniel saying to this man? How can the doctor not want to meet the rest of the family, talk to my husband and our other children? How can someone with purported negative personality changes occurring be taken at face value? There's no advocacy group for the family members of the mentally ill to go to for support and help during times such as this. There's no place for me to go and tell my views and what I'm seeing because the doctor has shut me out. Being not of the mental health world, I have no idea of anything I can do to shelter my family. If I push back on the doctor, he holds all of the power and isn't afraid to use it.

I find myself praying and asking God to keep my son sheltered from harm as he is around people selling drugs. I pray and ask God to keep my son sane with all of these toxins he's poisoning his system with daily. I know with everything in me that I have to get Daniel away from this psychiatrist. I now believe in my heart this doctor became a psychiatrist because he has his own emotional issues behind why he went into psychiatry. How can I get Daniel away from this man and bring back some sanity into the decisions that are made? I'm afraid if I pull Daniel out of Dr. Donovan's care, he'll call Child Protective Services and Daniel will be put into the foster care system. He won't survive long in his fragile state being isolated with strangers in the system. No one loves Daniel as much as his family and more harm than good will occur if this happens. I know Daniel won't live long if he's removed from us. We're walking through a nightmare, confronted by a maze of blocked corridors with no support.

God answers prayer in ways that are sometimes subtle, but life impacting. Leonard's work changes medical coverage and Dr. Donovan is no longer a Preferred Provider. I can hardly believe my eyes as I read the new insurance information and holding my breath check the listing of preferred providers. I feel an immense swelling of relief to have a route out of this doctor's grip that will keep us from being questioned. Now I need to find a good doctor that will help us heal Daniel. One where we're a team and the doctor doesn't divide us. One where we mutually work towards the outcome of Daniel's well-being. He'll need to see a doctor within our new network and I need to be sure this new doctor is one that sees Daniel being helped by a team which includes his family. My heart is uplifted for the first time in many months. I pray for God to help us locate a great doctor that will 'first, do no harm.'

CHAPTER SEVEN:

# Keep My Son from Destroying our Family

———◆———

*There is a sacredness in tears. They are not the mark of weakness, but of power. They speak more eloquently than ten thousand tongues. They are the messengers of overwhelming grief, of deep contrition, and of unspeakable love.*
*Washington Irving*

A family entering this trauma for the first time is dependent upon the medical psychiatric team to help bring their loved ones back to how they were before the illness. When the family finds themselves blamed with no ability to communicate and with their hands tied, they are not in a position to help the ill person. The old school way of thinking is that the mother is the cause of their child's mental illness. I'm stunned to find a doctor moving and working in this psychiatric model in the mid-1990s. I can't begin to talk about the trauma I feel being blamed for making my son sick, a child I gave my whole life to. I didn't return to work after my maternity leave following his birth because I didn't want a stranger watching and raising my child. I didn't want to risk the potential lack of love and caring. I was happy to walk away from my career and stay home with my children for 14 years. Now I am being blamed for raising my child horribly. I am destroyed, and my mind won't stop trying to find whatever it is I'm blamed for, since the doctor gave me no reasons. I'm at the mercy of a stranger who really knows nothing about our home life and makes no effort to know us. Judgment is raining down on us with no recourse or avenue for appeal. It was hard to stand strong in the face of the onslaught. I call my dad from time to time to touch base and find my center again. I can't imagine going through this without love and support from family members.

I'm excited to find a care provider at Grace Center by the name of Dr. Brian Pershall. From the very beginning the experience is different. Dr. Pershall wants me at the psychiatric sessions and if I'm not able to get away from work, he calls me and puts me on speaker phone. He talks about what Daniel shares and he asks me, "Do you have any items you want to talk about?" He wants to know how I think Daniel is doing during the week.

The turn-around in Daniel's care is amazing. He isn't able to weave a tale and get away with it without a counterbalance from the family. It helps keep him accountable and honest. No longer is he able to lie with impunity and without redress. How I wish everyone dealing with mental illness could have a doctor like this, one that knows it takes everyone to keep the person well. It isn't just done in isolation, but with a full accounting. I feel an immense relief. The ground feels like it's stabilizing under my feet and I'm beginning to think this might work and we might get Daniel well. I don't move in fear of the state knocking on my door anymore. I believe that maybe we can save Daniel.

During the years leading up to his graduation from high school, Daniel falls in with a crowd at high school that is messing around with alcohol, drugs, and Satanism. It's a cultural fad to dress in black, wear trench coats, and look gothic. Whenever Daniel can get his hands on alcohol and cigarettes, he sneaks off and drinks after school at someone's home. This is also the time in 1996, when a school shooting occurs in Moses Lake, Washington, by fourteen-year-old Barry Loukaitis.[viii] It's such an unusual event the entire country is discussing this sad scenario. I'm thinking to myself, "This could have been our family." When I see a picture of Barry, I am stunned at how much he looks like my son. He has those same vacant eyes. I wonder what his family members tried to do to get help. I remember back to the day when I walked into Daniel's room to find him loading his rifle, practicing for speed. It was at the same time as Barry Loukaitis was going through his own mental illness a few hours away from here. We could have so easily been in the same circumstance with our family murdered and people at school being victimized. Daniel became sick at this exact age and had I not aggressively fought for him in the system, he probably would've fallen through the cracks and became an even more withdrawn, angry loner. I shudder to think what would've happened if Daniel was stripped from us and sent into foster care without his family.

I wonder about parenting triggers that might have driven Barry to kill and I decide to have a conversation with my husband to ask him to change his approach with Daniel. I feel that Leonard's tough approach to parenting is going to push Daniel farther away. He believes Daniel's behavior is normal teenage behavior, and if Daniel just stops being a lazy kid and tries to apply himself, everything will be okay. He isn't seeing what I'm seeing and I can't make him understand what I think is going on. I know this can cause serious problems for our marriage, but I am trying to think of anything I can to will help bring less friction and stress to our home during this time. Leonard honors my request and stops trying to change Daniel's behavior through tough talk. It puts a huge burden on my shoulders to be the only one to manage the illness with Daniel and his medical psychiatric team, but I think it's for the best for now.

During the summer of 1997 my father has a bad car accident which damages his lungs and causes pleurisy. This car wreck leads to a worsening of his breathing and kicks his emphysema into high gear. Leonard and I decide to move my dad in to live with us and Daniel is excited. As my dad's breathing worsens over the ensuing months, we decide he needs more care than we can give him and we move him to an assisted living apartment. Daniel spends three to four nights a week at my dad's apartment, and is close to him. It's nice seeing the connection and closeness between the two of them. I find this bond helps Daniel make better choices and he decides to stop smoking because he sees the damage done to his grandpa. I'm thrilled and my dad is too. Their relationship stays strong and the years pass with Daniel staying pretty stable.

In the spring of 1999, Daniel and I go to Richard Wilkinson, M.D., in Yakima, Washington, to see if he can find any health issues which may be causing Daniel's mental health problems, hoping he might be able to help remedy the issues. Dr. Rick works on total body wellness; he looks at the whole system and works on the body in an integrative, functional manner. He discovers Daniel has a major food allergy to milk and we need to keep him off of anything containing it. He also begins nutrient therapy with Daniel, working on building up his body's nutrition. He adds in supplements to address a well-rounded approach to his diet. He puts Daniel on a solid multivitamin, vitamin B150, vitamin D, and probiotics. Daniel's improving steadily while also on his psychiatric medications. After a time, Dr. Rick slowly starts lowering his psychiatric medications while we're adding in supplementation. We eventually stop almost all of his psychiatric medications. It's nice to see Daniel happy and improving.

In June 2000, Daniel graduates from high school and for a graduation gift, his dad and I send him to London, England, with a high school friend. He has a great time and everything goes very well. I'm beginning to think maybe we're on to something and Daniel might recover his old self. After Daniel returns from London, Dr. Rick thinks he will have us add Inositol to his supplements because it has been shown to be very helpful with mental health issues. I start Daniel on the nutrient one evening and within hours we lose all the gains we made during the previous months. He becomes hyper, angry, agitated, anxious, sleepless, and paranoid. I'm shocked at the rapid change in Daniel after just one dose and call the doctor the very next morning.

Dr. Rick says, "Daniel is too fragile and you need to really work with his psychiatric team to get and keep him stable. I'm not comfortable with Daniel as a patient any longer and you should keep with the psychiatrist in town."

It's such a let-down because I really thought we were on to something. I understand Dr. Rick's hesitancy because if this goes south and we're harmed, he will potentially bear scrutiny and condemnation from the system. We had the old Daniel back with us during the time Dr. Rick pursued nutrients, but there must be something else going on that we need to address…if we only knew what it was. I wonder what about Inositol triggered the problem and why?

It's amazing that during these last five years Daniel is able to complete high school and also earn his Associate of Arts degree from college just one quarter after graduating high school. Having a good psychiatrist and teamwork is a game changer. Daniel really is an intelligent person and he works really hard at his classes. The Running Start Program is an incredible way for high school students to earn college credit while still in high school. Daniel takes advantage of the program and does well. It's impressive that through his psychosis and psychiatric medication, he's able to earn a college degree and finish high school by the age of 19. We're all so proud of him that he can work through the haze of prescription psychiatric medications and focus enough to learn and test.

By the fall of 2000, my dad dies from the complications of emphysema and this devastates both Daniel and me. We spend evenings talking about my dad and how impactful his life was on us. He had such a grounding influence and a calming spirit. There was no father as empowering and loving as my dad. He was always in my corner encouraging and building me up, making me believe anything was possible. I remember thinking that I hope Daniel makes it through this loss, as it is leaving such a huge hole from such a remarkable man. I'm watching Daniel closely and praying for the best. I stay by his side and am always available to talk and listen. I am sad to see him go almost immediately back to smoking cigarettes after my dad's death. I'm really surprised as he stopped smoking for three years while my dad was here with us. He saw what it looked like to suffer from emphysema and watched it take my dad's life, but I guess the sadness and loss is too much for Daniel to handle and smoking calms him down.

Daniel decides he wants to continue college, so Leonard, Daniel and I visit the University of Idaho because they have a good science and engineering program. We walk around checking out the chemistry lab and the campus layout. Daniel likes what he sees and applies. He's accepted. Leonard puts money down and reserves Daniel's spot. As the weeks goes by we can see Daniel become more and more anxious. Is it the loss of my dad or the stress of heading off to college?

He comes to me and tells me, "I can't cope with going away to the University. I know the stress will be more than I can handle."

In our weekly visit with Dr. Pershall, he also confirms that sending Daniel off to the University would be a poor decision. I am proud of how insightful Daniel is of his inability to cope in certain situations and let us know it's not in the cards right now.

Unfortunately, regardless of all our hard work and efforts to keep Daniel sane, he begins hearing voices and seeing demonic visions again.

"I'm hearing children chanting to me in my bedroom," he lets me know. "They are singing and repeating horrible things, they're not sweet nursery rhymes."

In the hopes that just changing his environment might help, we move Daniel to another upstairs bedroom where this traumatic event hasn't occurred yet, hoping he can sleep. We find him sleeping less and less as the months continue because he can't silence the voices and the singing children. He's starting to get dark circles under his eyes and his hygiene is rapidly deteriorating. I can't get him to change his clothes or bathe and he wears the same outfit for weeks on end. The smell is bad and his appearance is shocking.

# CHAPTER EIGHT:

## Keep My Son Sane

————◆————

*Every man has a sane spot somewhere.*
*Robert Louis Stevenson*

In the fall of 2000, Leonard takes Daniel to our pastor, Mark Samuels, to discuss our situation and see if his faith-based viewpoint will help educate us of the events that are occurring.

Daniel tells Mark, "I invited Loci the demon of war into me and all my great strength and all the positive stuff in my life is coming from him." Daniel also tells Mark he's reading the Satanic Bible. He goes on to tell Mark where he can find the book in the outskirts of town.

Mark tells us he asked Daniel if he could speak to the demon and Daniel's personality changed. Mark said he spoke to the demon Loci and Daniel needs an exorcism. Later, he went out to the location Daniel described earlier in the day and found the Satanic Bible right where Daniel said he left it. Mark burned the book.

After the session between Daniel and Mark, my husband calls to tell me what Mark thought about their session. When I arrive home in the afternoon with Karis, we find Daniel crawling around on the living room floor meowing like a cat and saying, "Here pussy, pussy." He's laughing hysterically.

In stunned silence, I turn to Karis and say, "Go grab your backpack because we need to go to a dentist appointment." This is an excuse to get us both out of the house and safe until Leonard gets home. Karis looks at me confused. I look her in the eyes and say again, "Go grab your backpack."

As Karis and I drive down the road, fleeing Daniel, I know I have to go back home because Daniel is really sick and needs me. I can't abandon him when he's at his sickest. I wish I had family in town where I could drop Karis off to keep her away from our home, but I don't. I'm hesitant to bring friends into the situation. I turn the car around and head back to our home. When Karis and I get back to the house, Daniel is gone. I just know he's going to commit suicide. My mind starts taking off on its own tangent, imagining every horrible thing it can. I just don't know how I can survive this if my son takes his own life. I spend the entire night awake in the living room in front of the fireplace just praying God will keep my son alive, and that he won't commit suicide. I am not able to sleep, and I just stare into the fireplace and replay the afternoon over and over in my head. I feel like I have really let him down, and by running away I left him to his demons. I know we move in the moment and we don't always get a redo. This is one of those moments and I'm hoping the outcome isn't devastating.

Suicide is a very real fear I have for Daniel. It causes me to weigh each word I am going to speak carefully before the words leave my mouth. Words can be so damaging, and I don't want to be the motivation for his death. The odds are drastically higher for people suffering from Bipolar disorder, which is Daniel's current diagnosis.[ix] This night is a long sorrowful affair for me, as I pray, "Please don't let there be a knock on my door from the police." As the sun is rising, Daniel comes rushing back into the house.

He comes up to me with eyes all glossy and he's frantically asking me, "Are you okay?" I'm standing in front of the refrigerator getting some water when he runs in.

He tells me, "I fell asleep at a friend's house and woke up and saw Satan and he was taunting me saying he's going to torture and rape you, and there isn't anything I can do to prevent it from happening and if I interfere, I'll be next." He's certain this is really happening and expected to find the scene occurring.

Daniel's really upset and shaking. He describes Satan's face as pure evil, and says, "Satan will not stop until you're hurt or dead." He's talking really fast and he's sure I'm in danger. I hug him tight, and tell him, "I am okay and God is keeping me safe and nothing happened to me in the night."

I respond firmly, "I love you and everything is okay. We're gonna be okay." I'm looking him in the eyes which are wild with fear and panic. He slowly begins to calm down and his agitation starts to abate. The frantic look in his eyes is leaving and I'm so sad he's caught in this illness because the trauma for him is as real as it is for me. I can't imagine this reality in his mind and I am suddenly sympathetic to why the mentally ill commit suicide to stop the pain.

This same morning, I talk with Daniel about heading out to his normally scheduled psychiatric appointment and he tells me, "I'm not going because the government controls the facility and they'll keep me there forever."

"It's just a clinic run by the local Catholic Church and not the Federal Government," I explain. I convince Daniel to go to the Grace Center for his scheduled appointment and I contact my husband so he can come with us. I feel such relief to have Leonard along because he helps me feel calm. He'll also get to see how the appointment goes and add his input when he feels ready. Leonard is increasingly concerned about Daniel's erratic behavior.

After the appointment starts, we tell his case manager, Bonnie, about the events of the last week and last night. We let her know about the satanic hallucinations and voices that are taking over Daniel's day.

Bonnie asks Daniel, "Tell me about Satan and Loci and their plans to hurt your mom. Do you really believe you see them and hear them?"

Daniel, looking all glassy eyed and strung out, replies, "Yes, they're real and I see and hear them all the time. I'm sure they want to hurt my mom. If I'm not careful and watchful, they will rape her."

After visiting awhile with Daniel, Bonnie gives him the option, "Put yourself in inpatient care at the psychiatric hospital for seventy-two hours, or if I admit you against your will, the stay can be as long as ten days."

Daniel's swift to reply, "I'm not sick, and the voices are real, as real as you are right now. I don't need to be in the hospital."

"You are sick, and we need to help make you well again. You really need to check yourself in for care." Bonnie can see him becoming agitated so again she reiterates, "If you don't agree to an inpatient stay at the hospital, you'll find that your forced inpatient stay, which will be against your will, will end up being longer."

"If I let you put me in the hospital, I'll never get out because the government controls everything and they won't ever let me leave." Daniel is adamant in his beliefs.

Bonnie gently lets Daniel know, "The government doesn't control this facility and as soon as you're stable we'll release you."

After a lot of negotiating and questions, Daniel chooses to admit himself. His first inpatient stay begins this afternoon at nineteen years of age, five years into our mental health journey. Bonnie leaves the room to go set up his inpatient bed, and coordinate the doctor and insurance coverage. She leaves my husband and me in the room with Daniel, who looks like we just sold him down the river to an unknown future, from which he's frightened he may never return.

He keeps telling me, "I told you this place is government controlled; they're going to keep me. I told you." He looks at me with an expression that tells me I betrayed him and put him up to this, knowing they'll never let him out.

"We'll come each day to see you, and you'll be released again, I promise," I tell Daniel. He just looks at me with distrust in his eyes.

My husband interjects, "Please just work with the doctors and comply with the medication changes. I know they can help if you'll let them. Please rest and work on getting better."

Daniel doesn't trust me anymore, and it's obvious he thinks I'm the enemy, but he seems to hear Leonard. A resignation spreads over Daniel and he goes silent as we wait for Bonnie to return for him. I keep reiterating, "We love you and will always be here for you; we aren't leaving you alone," but his eyes aren't focusing anymore, he's gone inside where he's preoccupied with whatever the voices are whispering to him at the moment.

I have such a profound sense of relief but my husband cries as they lead Daniel away. I think to myself, "This is the first moment where Leonard realizes Daniel truly has a psychiatric illness and this isn't just teenage trouble." Now I know my husband is starting to get it, to realize there's a definite psychiatric disorder going on, and he'll be a great help as we move forward with Daniel's care. Neither my husband nor I ever behaved like Daniel in our teen years or experienced this type of behavior first-hand. We have no tools to know how to parent during this phase. We were going off gut instinct these last five years.

Leonard is an awesome dad, he loves Daniel and wants him alive and well too. He's proactive and moves quickly to find remedies to problems. I feel such relief to know he's now going to be able to lift a lot of the load off my shoulders. Seeing Leonard cry as they lead Daniel away breaks my heart, but at the same time it gives me a huge sense of relief knowing that Leonard is now getting it and I won't be walking this alone anymore. It's a great day for me, and I leave the facility with such hope that the medical team will come up with a plan to recover Daniel and return him back to us.

I tell Leonard, "I'm relieved Daniel is going inpatient because he'll be safe and I won't have to worry about him for a couple days. He won't have access to anything to harm himself and maybe the psychiatric team will find an answer, or the right drug combination."

While Daniel is being led away to his first inpatient hospital stay, his younger brother Tyler is in his sophomore year at university and Karis is fourteen years old. Such a startling difference in outcomes and such a tragedy our brilliant son is now in a locked ward awaiting psychiatric care. Sometimes life doesn't make much sense. Our family has been through such a hard time these past five years and it's taking a toll. Tyler is pulling away physically from his brother because of his behavior and Karis looks on wondering what's going on. Her brother is getting worse by the year and nothing is helping. As an adult, I have a hard time processing what we're experiencing. I can only imagine how hard this is for Karis. None of her other peers are having these kinds of issues in their families, and there really isn't anyone in her group of friends that can help her come to terms with what's happening in our family. It's a very lonely place to be.

Leonard lets our pastor know about Daniel's inpatient stay at Grace Center. His response is, "I'm not surprised at the turn of events since I confronted Daniel yesterday; I figure I triggered something in his mind."

I am still not sure how to process the church's approach of needing an exorcism. I know something is wrong, but I'm at a loss as to how to move forward. I don't know how to logically move on if we buy into this demon possession theory and all it implies. I am afraid when I'm in Daniel's presence and I know he's fixated on Satan and demons. Although possession doesn't ring true to me, I want to be open to anything that will bring my son back from the brink of insanity.

At the hospital, Daniel is assigned an inpatient psychiatrist named Dr. Harvey. Leonard and I meet with Dr. Harvey for the first time to discuss Daniel's psychiatric condition, what the plan is for the path forward, and to allow him to inform us of the potential mental health impacts for our son.

"Each time Daniel has another psychotic episode," Dr. Harvey tells us, "he'll suffer more brain injury and this will damage the neurotransmitter receptors, flattening them out so they won't work as well. After each subsequent episode, we have the potential to get less and less of your son back on the other side of the psychotic break."

This is chilling news to hear. I haven't considered the long term repercussions of psychotic breaks over the years. I can't wrap my mind around losing Daniel piece by piece as episode after episode unfolds. It seems like we're a prisoner to the mental health fragility of Daniel's mind.

Dr. Harvey continues, "Learn how to watch for important signs of upcoming issues and potential psychotic breaks around the corner, and try to prevent them from escalating to the point where Daniel will need to go inpatient for care. If we can cut off the psychosis from becoming full blown, we may be able to get him back on some form of stable footing before it gets too hard to retrieve him again."

"Our son believes he has invited a demon into himself and he's engrossed with Satan," I inform the doctor. "Is this a true statement? Have you seen this before? What do we make of it?" The questions just tumble out of my mouth. Trauma and tortured thoughts which need settling. Are we safe? How do we parent this?

"This is all a part of the disease process where he's caught in his delusions and hallucinations," Dr. Harvey assures me, "Your son believes they're true, but they are not and we need to reach him in his illness and help him."

Leonard and I visit Daniel each evening while he's at the hospital. The first time we enter the psychiatric ward is frightening. Never having been in a locked facility before, it's uncomfortable to know we won't be getting out unless a nurse with a key is available. There are quite a few people waiting to be buzzed into the locked hospital. We stand outside the facility and hit the button alerting the nurses to our presence.

"Diane and Leonard Borders to see Daniel Borders." They buzz us in and we join the group which is congregating in the waiting room.

A nurse comes out to talk to the group before she leads us through the locked door. She tells us the rules for visiting the locked psychiatric facility. No shoestrings, no belts, all clothing must be checked by a staff member to ensure all articles of clothing are approved. If we have any packages, the staff will need to go through everything piece by piece.

"A smoking area is in the center of the ward," she says, "and many of the patients are out there smoking. You are not allowed to go into the patient rooms, but are able to sit in the common area to visit."

I'm nervous as we pass through the locked door and enter the hospital ward the first night. All of the patients are sitting in the designated enclosed atrium area smoking cigarettes. Some visitors take seats on the couches inside and wait for their loved ones to finish smoking on the other side of the glass. It's amazing how much relief the patients receive from smoking and they come back in visibly more calm. Leonard and I go outside and join Daniel while he smokes.

"Mom and I love you very much and hope everything is going okay as you settle in," Leonard says. I agree with my husband and tell Daniel I'm glad he's getting his medications adjusted and I hope he feels better soon. Everyone is sitting with their loved ones and trying to make connections with them and give them hope. It's such a sad and conflicted place to be. You feel bad your loved one is there, but you also feel they're safer there getting help.

The nurses and doctors are there with us, intermingling with the patients and their families. It's a time to connect with the psychiatric team and ask questions, and I'm grateful for their presence. During Daniel's stay, he looks forward to one particular visitor. He's dating a young lady name Barb. She's a gentle person who brings out the good in Daniel. She's quite a bit younger than him but isn't put off or afraid that he went inpatient in the psychiatric hospital. She comes to visit him and stands by his side. It amazes me to see her not walk away. She doesn't need to invest herself in a situation like this, why does she stay? It's soothing to me to know she's by his side and it gives him hope.

During the week while Daniel is in treatment and visiting hours are in progress, we find ourselves ushered into a room and locked in with the other visitors while the staff takes a violent patient to a padded room. This is an unsettling feeling knowing some of the patients can be dangerous and need to be restrained. We've been so sheltered in our existence up until this time. It's an innocence I wish our family still possessed.

During one evening visit, a young lady is sitting in the sofa area and is singing a beautiful song to God. Her voice is amazing. She turns her eyes to heaven and sings with everything inside of her. As the minutes go by, the singing becomes louder and louder and louder, until everything else is drowned out and people can't hear each other talking. She never averts her eyes from heaven and is enthralled by what she's experiencing. It seems like she can look straight to heaven and see God and angels. A nurse comes over and asks the young lady to come with her and they take her to her room. A short while later, after an injection, the young lady comes back and sits on the sofa. This time she's calm and holding a Bible on her lap and she is reading God's word.

I find myself wishing Daniel had the angelic form of mental illness instead of the demonic. When I meet with Dr. Harvey the next day, I ask him about the satanic verses God aspect of what I am seeing.

He tells me, "Frequently the mentally ill present with direction and voices which are either demonic or angelic."

I think to myself that I'd prefer the angelic version of mental illness because at least the message is one of grace and love. However, as time goes on, I learn the mentally ill believe God speaks to them and can ask them to commit horrific acts in the name of God. How does a mentally ill person withstand directions from

God and not act? At least with Daniel, I can come back with responses like, "We know in the end who wins, and it isn't Satan." In this way I can try and dispel the mesmerizing influence of the voices in Daniel's head by a force more powerful than Satan.

As mental illness grips my family, it makes me more aware of mental illness in our communities and I'm drawn to stories of real life tragedy involving the mentally ill. I thank God for keeping my son safe and alive so far, and I continually pray for His guidance as we move through this psychiatric maze. As I read the stories, I'm gripped by the fact no one seems willing to step forward and do the hard stuff of putting these people in inpatient, long-term care. The mentally ill have rights that keep them from this care. So much of the time they don't see they are ill and have no concept of the fact they are sick. This is called anosognosia, which is a condition where people with serious mental health issues are unaware of their own illness.

In 1983, Bruce Blackman, a twenty-two-year-old paranoid schizophrenic, slaughters his six family members in Vancouver, Canada. Blackman suffers from the belief the world is coming to an end and he has to do something about it. Killing his family members is his way of preserving them forever.[x] In 2001, Andrea Yates murders her five children by following commands she hears from God and Satan. She believes Satan can't control her and her children anymore once she kills them.[xi] In 2005, Sheilla Shea stabs her six-year-old to death in front of her other children and then tries to kill herself by stabbing herself in the chest three times. Sheila suffers from paranoid schizophrenia and believes people are coming to hurt her and her children. She thinks by killing her children and herself, she's protecting them from the evil intentions of others. She later tries to hang herself while in jail by shredding a bed sheet and wrapping it around her neck.[xii]   On Halloween evening of 2014, Derek Ward, thirty-five years old, kills and beheads his mother Patricia, kicking her head across the street before throwing himself in front of a train.  He had been off of his medication for four days and his mother was trying to get him into care.[xiii]

These are just a few of the stories which flood our papers and community's day in and day out.  It's time to wake up and repair our mental health system to protect our families, and get care for those who don't even realize they are mentally ill.  Surely, mothers don't kill their children and sons don't kill their families, and yet it's in the news every day.  Most of us go about our business unaffected by the mentally ill.  However, for those of us who struggle with loved ones who are ill, we live with this situation each day.  These events remind me we're walking a fragile line between safety and sanity.  In an instant, my family can find ourselves in a story much the same.  We need to educate the public and ourselves about mental illness and the devastating consequences when severe mental illness goes untreated.  Our mental health system in the United States is failing our loved ones and our families by allowing them to refuse treatment until they're deemed a danger to themselves or others.  This is a twisted way to go about helping people.

It's at this time we realize we may need to adjust the hopes and dreams we hold as parents for Daniel and his future.  Who knows where this course is taking him and our family.  Daniel also knows changes are happening to his mind and he's finding it harder and harder to read, comprehend, and regurgitate data on a test.  His brain is failing him.  I'm sure it's hard on him to see his younger brother head off to university, pursuing his future, while he struggles with his daily existence.  This is not the plan Daniel had in mind for his life.

Daniel's case manager, Bonnie, encourages us during this inpatient stay to get Daniel designated as disabled through Social Security. My husband and I don't want to do this because we have insurance that will help us take care of the medical bills. Bonnie speaks to us at length over the week about the possibility that Daniel will outlive us and that our other two children may not be able to care for him. With Daniel designated as disabled, the social security system will step in and make sure he has a roof over his head, medical care, and food on his table. We initiate the paperwork and through the process they tell us the system always denies everyone, then we'll have to file for a reconsideration of Daniel's case. The whole process can take up to two years. Of course, they tell us we can hire a lawyer to help speed the process up. We decide to just let the system run its course and see what happens. I'm amazed this government system is tolerated, but I guess no one has any other options, so the federal government and the state get can away with the ineffective process.

I frequently tell Daniel, "Don't give up, the medical community and researchers are always working on new medications and every ten years there's usually a huge leap in understanding. Eventually we'll stumble upon an answer which will make a profound difference." Soon we'll know more about how to tackle this illness and find out what's behind the erosion of his mental capacity that's so horribly impacting his life. As depressed as I am about seeing Daniel go from a brilliant young man to one lost in his own internal turmoil, I can hardly imagine the trauma and pain he pushes through each day. I know he has to persevere through his journey and I pray each day the Lord will heal Daniel and bring him back to the whole person he was. I need to unconditionally love him, and to do anything else is to fail him when he's at his weakest. When the stability of life is gone, there's just love for one another. We are all we have; we're one family. God will give us strength and help us endure. At the same time, I don't understand how we're already five years in and no healing is happening and on a downhill slide with apparent limited help.

At the end of the week of his first inpatient stay, we take Daniel home with us on adjusted medications and pray for the best. I hope Daniel will see God's grace through me, and learn to forgive me from what he sees as a betrayal when he was admitted to the hospital. I know our other two kids are frightened of his behavior and this is alienating them, but I also see them protecting and encouraging Daniel too. I remember Karis coming home from school one day so offended by her friends talking poorly about the mentally ill. After hearing about the story and her pain, I let her know they are speaking from a place of ignorance.

"They have not walked in your shoes," I tell her, "they can't know the impact of mental illness. When you feel ready, you can help teach them the reality of being faced with a mentally ill loved one." I am trying to encourage her spirit. She's growing through hardship and I know this will form an amazing young lady full of compassion, grace, and love. I hate to see her learn through fire, but sometimes that's how we learn the most and understand things more deeply. Daniel is still her big brother with good memories. I'll always remember Karis in her bumble bee costume as a little girl, acting like she's going to sting Daniel, chasing him all over the house and him feigning fright at the bee. She gets him down on the sofa and gets on top of him and attempts to bite him. This awesome scene forever keeps me smiling and hopeful. Karis adores her brother and instinctively knows we can't abandon him now.

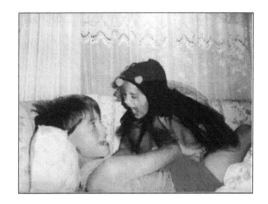

# CHAPTER NINE:

## Keep My Son Stable

———◆———

*Do not be anxious about tomorrow, for tomorrow will be anxious for itself.*
*Let the day's own trouble be sufficient for the day.*
*Matthew 6:34*

In 2001, my husband helps Daniel get a job at a bookstore. He thought this would be a great fit for Daniel because he's always loved books. He began reading at age 5, and has quite a collection of books. Daniel decides to take the job and is assigned to work the cash register. He enjoys helping the customers. When he isn't working at his bookstore, he often goes to another nearby bookstore to browse through their books. It seems odd that he doesn't just shop at his bookstore where he gets discounts, but he says, "I'm just browsing, not buying. Shopping at my bookstore after I get off work makes me feel like I never leave the job." It's nice to see him heading off to work and out in the community.

His days are falling into a rhythm at his job, but as summer progresses I can tell something is changing, and I am trying to do as Dr. Harvey suggests and keep my eyes open for signs that his medication is no longer working well. He's beginning to seem off, and agitated more frequently, and I can see him standing at the living room window watching cars pass by. He's becoming more paranoid as the months go by.

Unfortunately, in the summer of 2001, as is now a common occurrence, Daniel goes to the other bookstore to browse and get out of the house. Daniel is looking through their books and notices the employees are following him and watching him. In his fragile state, this causes his paranoia to escalate and he begins acting strangely inside the store. He starts walking around the store staring at people, while they are following and watching him, and he's imagining they're thinking and planning something. Unbeknownst to Daniel, apparently there were two young men that just robbed the store while Daniel was there. The workers think Daniel may be a part of the team as they all arrived at the same time. The employees call the police and then keep their eyes on Daniel, following him around until they arrive.

The police forcibly put Daniel on the ground and place handcuffs on his wrists as they ask him questions. Of course, this only heightens his agitation to a point where his behavior is quite paralyzing. He has such a fear of the police and government and this is playing right into his worst nightmare and his paranoia. When the police check Daniel's ID and find he has money in his wallet and a nice Toyota Camry outside, they let him go.

The police let Daniel up off of the floor, remove the handcuffs, and the bookstore manager tells Daniel, "You are no longer allowed to shop in this store." They do not arrest our son, but he's quite humiliated. Leonard happens to be out of town on business when this transpires, and when I tell him what occurred, he's furious. This is the last thing we need with Daniel already afraid of the police and starting to have paranoia issues again.

Leonard contacts the police and complains to them about Daniel's treatment. He finds out that in the chaos of the takedown of Daniel, and Daniel not thinking properly afterward, the police forgot to give him back his driver's license. The police officer, in coordination with my husband, meets with Daniel at his workplace to apologize and return his license. Leonard makes sure Daniel's manager is present for the apology in case the two stores have any contact.

I am not sure if this whole scenario impacts Daniel's mental state, but it isn't long after his hostile treatment that he abruptly quits his job. This comes as such a surprise to us, as he has the most sales of discount cards and enjoys working behind the counter. His manager phones me to let me know that he quit.

"Daniel was working his shift at the bookstore last evening and everything seemed normal. All of the sudden he disappeared. We were looking for him and couldn't find him." She tells me, "I put a person on his cash register and as we were working we found a note inside a book." The note said, I'm quitting work to pursue my interest in fashion. Books no longer interest me.

I am stunned to say the least. The manager goes on, "He put the note inside a book, letting it stick out of the top, and left it right next to the cash register. He just walked out of the store. No discussion. No warning. He just disappeared during his shift."

"I'm surprised at what he's done, but he's having some health issues." I tell her.

"With the state Daniel is in, we can no longer employ him, even if he changes his mind." She wishes us luck with Daniel and wishes him the best and goes on to tell me she enjoyed having Daniel on staff.

We are starting on another downward spiral and it doesn't seem like there's anything we can do to slow this down. I had high hopes for the medication change after his hospital stay, but they aren't having the proper effect. Daniel's becoming anxious, angry, unfocused, is not sleeping, and is paranoid. Each month we limp along trying to make the best of his situation. He's rudderless and drifting. Everyone else is moving forward and making plans while we're just thankful Daniel is still breathing and walking. It's amazing how little you come to expect good things to happen for your loved one who is fighting mental illness. You find yourself happy they're alive and that is the marker you place against everything.

By December of 2001, Daniel is seeing Dr. Pershall at the Grace Center on a regular basis. Dr. Pershall gives him the diagnosis of Schizoaffective, Bipolar Type. The following are notes from Dr. Pershall given to Daniel's pediatrician.

"Daniel states, for the most part, his moods have been more on the up side. His thoughts are going quick. His speech is quick. He denies any grandiose thoughts. He denies any thoughts of wanting to commit suicide, although he has flashes of death. He also denies any homicidal ideation. He goes to bed at 6 a.m. and wakes up at 10 a.m. His appetite is up and down. His energy is on the highest side.

He has thoughts of mass killers and has a fascination toward these individuals. He says he would not act out on these types of actions that these past killers engaged in.

He says that at night sometimes he sees flashes of people or sees a purple haze on the road when he is driving at night. He has some suspiciousness regarding criminals and law enforcement agents. He feels like they might say that he has done something wrong that he has not. He states that over the summer he was arrested at the bookstore for acting suspicious, but he had not committed a criminal act."

By February 2002, Daniel is admitted to the Grace Center on a voluntary basis due to his rapid decline into a psychotic state. Daniel's stay is scheduled for two weeks. He walks in to the hospital and says, "I need to be admitted because I'm drinking so heavily I know I'll die if I don't admit myself." The Grace Center calls me and tells me they don't really do it this way, but they'll keep him because he's so fragile. It probably helps that he's still on private insurance and they don't have to work the Medicaid system. We're still awaiting the ruling on Social Security Disability.

Grace Center admits him and spends time trying to address his drinking and help him to understand that drinking causes his medications to not work as well. He goes to group sessions and fills out his lesson sheets which try to teach him common sense information to help him choose well. Daniel tells them, "I won't drink anymore. I can see its bad for me." He tells them all of the right things and seems committed to not drink.

I'm hopeful and at work, I tell my friend Jody, "I think the drinking will stop."

She looks at me and says point blank, "There's no way this is over, Daniel will drink again."

This statement really shocks me and it stops me in my tracks. Jody has spent years working in the juvenile justice system and she's seen so much. Compared to her, I'm pretty sheltered and am looking for anything to hold on to. I tell myself to not get my hopes up and be on alert for signs of Daniel drinking again. Hearing Jody say this helps put the situation in perspective and realigns my hope to reality. I am hopeful, but I'm watchful. If he drinks I'll be prepared for the situation and not be so devastated. Thank goodness for friends that aren't afraid to speak the truth as they see it. At the end of the two weeks, Daniel is released on Risperdal and Lithium medication.

Fourteen months have gone by since Daniel applied for Social Security Disability and we finally hear back that he's approved. His medications are covered along with his visits to the doctor. Daniel still lives with us but we're relieved to know if something happens to us, there's a safety net to help him.

I spend many months researching nutritional support for people with schizoaffective disorder. I know somehow there's more to the story of Daniel's sudden illness, there has to be more going on at the cellular level that triggered his disorder. He was only fourteen years old when this hit out of nowhere, maybe it's somehow tied to the hormones of puberty, or how his body is able to process nutrition. It seems logical that there's some kind of cellular switch which kicks in causing everything to go haywire.

Through my research I find a product called True Hope Nutritional which works to heal the body through a nutrient therapy approach. Daniel is willing to give the supplements a try and we call True Hope to discuss how to implement their program. With the product on the way, we have hope this will bring him some relief. We spend time on the phone with their staff working out how to proceed. Daniel follows the dosing and is taking the supplements faithfully. We see a marked improvement in his depression and he seems less agitated and anxious. Every week Daniel fills out a log of how he feels in many different categories and we report back to True Hope via the phone. They work with their clients to make sure they're moving forward and having positive results. I am surprised to see an improvement and hopeful.

In August 2002, Daniel turns twenty-one and he begins drinking alcohol excessively. This causes him to stop following his medication plan and he also stops taking his True Hope supplements. The alcohol really messes up how his body uses the medication and how it absorbs nutrients. He's now prone to flushing his prescriptions down the toilet saying he doesn't need them anymore. When I point out to him the changes his choices are making in his health and how far he's regressing back into ill health, he responds, "I'm not you."

When you mix mental illness and addiction together you get an impossible situation. As time goes on, Daniel becomes a very mean drunk and quite ill. He loses his girlfriend Barb after he pushes her too far with his cruel words. She stood by him through a couple years, and a couple inpatient stays, but she can't withstand the effects of alcohol on his mental state. Barb is gone and I grieve her absence. During the early days after she leaves, Daniel calls her and leaves messages that talk about suicide followed by other messages condemning her for leaving him. I tell him he needs to back off and leave her alone because he can get in a lot of trouble if he continues threatening her.

"She can get a restraining order against you and this is something you don't need on your record," I tell him. "If you don't stop drinking then you are making your choice to lose Barb and choose alcohol." He can't walk away from the booze…he chooses alcohol.

As Daniel's mental deterioration continues, he finds himself once again in the mental hospital at the Grace Center. The doctors are having a hard time stabilizing him due to the effects of the alcohol in his system. It's causing his medication to not work correctly and makes correct dosing hard to figure out. Daniel says all the right words to the inpatient doctor but he has no intention of following their advice once he's released from care. During this third inpatient stay, Leonard and I again go every evening to let Daniel know we're standing beside him and want only the best for his future.

One evening when I go by myself, Daniel and I are visiting on the sofa when out of nowhere he tells me, "You have Munchausen by Proxy."

I burst out laughing and I am expecting him to smile but he's dead serious and distant. I can feel heat rising up through my body from my feet up to my head. I am overtaken by such incredulousness that I'm momentarily speechless. I look at him with confused eyes and I tell him, "If you think this is the future I want for myself, then you're mistaken. You have caused such chaos and misery in our family over the last seven years and everyone struggles with the outcome your behavior causes." Our family is heavily impacted by him and his unwillingness to stop drinking.

"I love you, but I don't know you anymore." I immediately stand up, pick up my purse, holding my tongue to stop the instinctual verbal lashing that I really want to do, and grab the nurse to ask her to let me out of the locked ward. From this moment on, I know I can never go see Daniel alone at the hospital. It seems whenever I'm alone with him, he'll say things to me to hurt and shock me. I don't understand why he's doing this and I don't know how to respond. I find myself stuffing down my responses to him and internalizing them. I am afraid if he knows what I really feel and think, it will cause him so much turmoil and self-loathing he'll want to commit suicide.

When Leonard and I arrive the next evening Daniel doesn't mention anything about our Munchausen conversation. It's been eating me up for the last 24 hours and it didn't mean a thing to him. I wonder if he even remembers.

"I had an IQ evaluation with Dr. Drew last night," Daniel is happy to let us know. "My intelligence measures in the top one half of one percent of the population." He's ecstatic and seems vindicated that he's perfectly normal and we're the ones with the mental issues. He continues, "You're trying to make me like you, and I'm not like you at all."

When we get home that evening I talk with Karis about our conversation. "Mom, I don't think this really happened. Dr. Drew is a doctor on television. I think this is a delusion Daniel is having and it's not real."

I immediately go on to the Grace Center provider network online looking to see if they have a Dr. Drew on staff and find they don't. I call my husband and Karis into the office and show them the physician listing. "Karis you're right. I can't believe it's not true." My husband and I were pulled into Daniel's delusion just that easily. He was so firm and lucid and clear on the entire IQ test. I sit here stunned and then find myself laughing. I am becoming harder and harder to shock. What's next in this cycle of mental illness? This episode is harmless but it also shows how Daniel is losing touch with reality and we're easily manipulated with lies that he totally believes are real.

In the psychiatric ward, it's hard to get used to the rules regarding no belts or shoe strings, nothing that Daniel can use to hurt himself or others. We bring Daniel flip flop sandals and he uses a rubber band to keep his pants up. Whenever I read stories about people who try to kill themselves while confined in jail or a psychiatric facility, I always wonder why they don't have the same rules enforced for their patients.

Daniel is released again with his medications adjusted. I've come to understand this will be a temporary fix and his meds will hold up only so long, then he'll be back in the hospital again. It seems like every eighteen months or so, we're back in the hospital with Daniel sicker than the previous visit. His mental health continues to deteriorate and we can't stop his alcohol abuse. The doctor from our first inpatient stay was right, each time we get Daniel handed back to us after a hospitalization, he isn't nearly as well as the time before. Damage is occurring within his brain and we're receiving a lesser version of our son with each discharge.

One blessing is the fact that Daniel has paranoia issues regarding law enforcement. At this early stage of mental illness, he's afraid to do anything that will break the law. In this way we're able to avoid the legal arrests for narcotics that plague so many other mentally ill patients. His drugs of choice are cigarettes and alcohol. Daniel can legally drink alcohol so we have limitations on preventing consumption. I take away his bank card so he can't get cash to purchase alcohol. Amazingly, he walks into his bank and show his driver's license to get cash out of his account so he has no need for the bank card. There are many times when I wish there was a law that allowed us to mark a driver's license with a symbol which would keep Daniel from buying alcohol due to his mental illness. We're caught in a predicament. Daniel needs his psychiatric medication to work in order to stop the delusions and hallucinations, but alcohol is hampering the medication from doing its jobs and we have no way to stop the purchase or theft of the substance.

Each night before I go to bed, I bring my purse upstairs and place it by my bedside. If I don't hide my money, Daniel will steal my cash to purchase alcohol. It's so strange to see him drink so heavily and never throw up. It's like he's building a tolerance and has to drink more and more to blackout which is his goal.

One day I ask him, "Why won't you work with us to stop drinking and get sober? You know your medication will work better if you don't drink alcohol. This may help with the delusions and hallucinations that are bothering you so much."

"Why would you want me sober to live through all of this and be completely aware? I drink to black out because this is the only way to quiet the voices." He replies. I'll never forget his response. I sit here for a moment and think to myself that I really have no appreciation for the turmoil Daniel lives in each and every day. To have voices crowding out your existence with negative comments and condemning, hateful threats all day long, every single day.

"Please hang in there and hopefully as time goes by we'll learn more about how to help you."

Daniel's excited to move out of our home and into an apartment he'll share with his friend Bob. I know he feels better about himself not living at home with us and we also feel relief that he seems happy with this new living arrangement. Daniel and Bob met at college and quickly became friends. We hope this arrangement works and Daniel will settle down and enjoy his new life.

However, Daniel's drinking escalates. When I go to bed at night, I have to turn the ringer off on my telephone so I won't be awakened by Daniel ranting and raving horrible comments to me. His messages are becoming more and more violent and rage filled. I save each message and ensure Daniel's doctor listens to them at each subsequent visit. I feel such guilt at turning off my phone because I'm sure one of these nights he may need me and I'll miss the call for help. However, I'm not getting any sleep and the phone calls are taking a toll on my health. I have to wake up at 5 AM to get ready for work and I can feel my stress level rising to an intolerable level. It's a horrible feeling when you see a voice message indicator from your son, and you know you'll be hit with an onslaught of hate filled incomprehensible babble. The real hell of Daniel's sickness continues to wash over our family and I'm at a loss for what to do. Just when I think things can't get any worse, I'm shocked and horrified with something new. I find Daniel tries hard to hide his behavior from everyone but me. It seems like he saves the horrible comments and threats just for me when he gets me isolated.

Days go by and we see Daniel less and less frequently. I only hear from Bob when Daniel gets out of control and too drunk. We have episodes where Bob calls me to come pick up Daniel and move him home.

On one such episode Daniel calls me and asks, "Come get me, I have to move home." I arrive to find Daniel has written all kinds of derogatory stuff on the walls with markers and is screaming and angry. I know I have to get him out of the apartment complex quickly or the police may be called by other worried residents. As I'm driving him home, I hold my breath and hope everything works out and he calms down. In the silence, Daniel blurts out incomprehensible words. I am so afraid of him at this point that I don't want to engage him in any way because he's drunk. I just want to get home without an incident since I'm all alone.

He keeps on mumbling words I can't understand and I look over at him and ask, "Can we just ride in silence?"

He replies with slurred speech, "Oh that's right, we don't want to talk about it."

If we can't stop the alcoholism, we can't stabilize the medication. If we can't stabilize both we can't hold any kind of meaningful conversations. I live in fear of speaking the wrong words, so I go mute and I stuff everything. I have no idea how to reach Daniel or engage him in any way. I don't want the rage I just saw at Bob's apartment to turn my way. Our existence has become a rollercoaster of moving Daniel in and out of our home. Bob keeps Daniel as long as he can tolerate the situation, but he has his limits and doesn't want to be forced out of the apartment because of Daniel's behavior. Each time this happens, there's no place for him to go but to the streets or back into our home.

# CHAPTER TEN:

## Keep My Son Resilient

———◆———

*Time discovers truth.*
*Lucius Annaeus Seneca*

Beginning in 2005, I spend a lot of time looking for any new research on mental illness and search for any new theories I can pursue as options in Daniel's care. I find a website by Amy Yasko, Ph.D., who is breaking new ground in the study of genetic mutations and the methylation pathway. As I am reading through her information and watching her videos, I'm struck by her discussion of the symptoms and issues Daniel is dealing with. I discover Dr. Yasko looks at thirty single nucleotide polymorphisms (SNPs) on the methylation pathway which she feels if addressed, a person can get their cell function working in a manner which will improve their health. She is looking for mutations in genetic allele pairs, which can affect the biochemistry of the body functions. Our genes are donated from mom and dad. You may receive a healthy non-mutated gene, or you may receive one mutated gene, or two mutated genes. It's the luck of the draw. I like to think of it as the old fashioned bingo games where the balls are popping up and down and all around in a huge box by the force of air. One by one they shoot up the tube and are selected at random. No control over which you'll get… a crap shoot.

Her information alludes to the fact that if no mutations are present, then the function at that SNP site is at 100%. One mutation and the SNP may be functioning at 60 to 70% of normal. Two mutations (one from mom and one from dad) may cause the SNP to only be working at 20 to 30% of normal. Mutations in the methylation SNP locations, if found to be double mutated, can greatly impact our health. Groups of many single mutations in a gene region may have decreased function equivalent to a double mutation. This situation can affect how the body is able to work. Each SNP site has a specific job to do, and if they are mutated, the job won't get done optimally. Dr. Yasko's blood test also includes her literature, diagrams, training materials, and a supplementation listing. Another company, 23andme, tests 600,000+ SNPs. They offer some information on health risks and ancestry, but they can't help with methylation and what it means, or teach someone how to proceed to address the mutation sites. However, it's a lot of raw data which could be useful in the future as more is learned about genetics and how they contribute to illness.

At this point in time, I can't afford to purchase either test but the idea of a genetic mutation causing Daniel's illness sounds intriguing. The idea of illness coming off of cellular function in the body just makes sense. Why don't we look at the single smallest denominator in our body and ensure these cells get exactly what they need to function? Instead of medicating the person with manmade synthetic prescription drugs, like antipsychotics which have their own serious side effects. Treatment can focus on repairing cellular function using nutrients, amino acids, enzymes, minerals, etc. and maybe the patient can progress to a lower dose of antipsychotics.

Time goes by quietly with Daniel sharing an apartment with Bob. Now and then Daniel shows up at the house and spends the night, but usually by the next morning he's gone again. It's a good time for me to spend reading and researching. Our family is busy with everyone off in different directions.

In 2007, Karis finishes her associate degree with straight A's and is off to a private university with an academic scholarship. We're really proud of her. At the same time, Daniel and I work on a psychosis profile we'll use to help us figure out when we're losing ground and when his medications are becoming ineffective again. This is a great idea suggested earlier to us by his inpatient doctor (Dr. Harvey) on one of his early stays at the Grace Center. I am a little on edge because it's been awhile since Daniel was in the hospital, so I'm feeling the need to work on this list and be ready and prepared.

The plan is while Daniel is lucid we'll create this list of symptoms associated with a worsening of his psychiatric condition which are specific to him. As we start seeing some of these symptoms occurring in his presentation, I can point to that symptom on his wall chart proving he recognized these negative symptoms when he was well and we'll get him in for help quickly. Hopefully he'll comply when faced with this evidence. It will help us try to make sure he doesn't hit a psychotic state again and end up with potential brain damage. For Daniel, his predominant issues are lack of hygiene because he rarely bathes, often wearing the same clothes for weeks without changing, paranoia, grandiose thinking, delusions, hallucinations, hearing voices, anger, mania/depressive swings, and seeing demons.

Early one morning I miss a call from Tyler. He's been rushed to the hospital for an emergency appendix operation. Tyler's in-laws are afraid to knock on our door in the middle of the night because they know my fear of a doorbell ringing, opening the door to the police, and being told Daniel is dead. Since I have my phone ringer off every night to avoid erratic phone calls from Daniel, I don't receive Tyler's voice message that he's in the hospital until I wake up at 5 am for work. As soon as I play the message, my husband and I immediately head to the hospital to be with Tyler.

It's sad our other two amazing children, Tyler and Karis, are always existing in this environment of sickness, shock, and fear. I'm sad for the pain they endure with all of the uncertainty and trauma that occurs around our family dealing with this mental illness. Mental illness affects the entire family, not just the ill person. Leonard and I try to give the kids our love and attention as equally as possible, but sometimes life has a way of placing obstacles in our paths.

As Daniel's illness progresses, I find the only way I can find peace and quiet for my mind, from all of the 'what if' scenarios, is to go to our church youth service on the week night. This is an amazing worship time with hundreds of youth, and I make sure to get there early so I can get a seat. It's always a packed house and I don't want to miss out on the time I can spend healing my soul. This is the time where I work on keeping myself grounded and keep myself from getting sucked into the vortex of mental illness. It helps calm my spirit and gives me hope. It may just be me, but when I turn to the church body, I feel like I spend too much time explaining the mental illness situation just to get hit back with, "It must be the devil," or "He needs to repent and have an exorcism," or "You must not have enough faith." I can't find the words to explain the situation. Having lived it for so many years and knowing all the nuances of mental illness, it can't be explained to someone quickly. They don't understand, can't understand, because even I can't grasp the situation, so I find myself not sharing our family turmoil with others. I recall that unless a person walks through a journey like this one, they can't empathize or relate to the struggle. I don't allow myself to be angry at their responses, I just know it comes from a place of ignorance.

If I didn't have my faith, I know I wouldn't have made it this far. I give my troubles and fears over to Christ and let him know I'm not strong enough, but I know he is. I ask Him to give me peace and protect me, guide me, lead me, and show me what I'm missing because if he isn't going to heal Daniel as I am asking, then He has to show me what my role will be in bringing my son back to sanity. I pray for wisdom to understand what I'm reading, and that Christ will open my mind to learn all that I need to know to tie the pieces together for Daniel.

One evening, I try attending a National Alliance on Mental Illness (NAMI) group. NAMI is a safe place for the wounded to gather. It's comforting to be with other people battling the same life issues. Mental illness in any family keeps people isolated and unwilling to trust anyone out of fear of being judged. During the meeting, I listen to a mom talk about her son and their fight with his mental illness. He's currently incarcerated in our local jail and when he finishes his time served, he'll immediately be placed under arrest again and serve another jail term to fulfill another sentence. She states that she's billed for his jail time because he's a minor and she's responsible for his fines. She's close to losing her home as the bills pile up from her mentally ill child's incarceration. This doesn't even sound right or just, surely she must be mistaken.

After the mother finishes her story, we have another guest speaker; a local judge who talks about the judicial system in our area and how they're working on creating a court for the mentally ill. The idea is that when a sick person is brought in to jail, they're evaluated and if the court finds they have a mental health issue, the court will divert them off to a separate mental health court. In this way, they can treat the person for their mental illness and release them back into the community when they're stable. Currently, the mentally ill are warehoused in our jails where their psychiatric needs aren't being met by the system, and their medications aren't being supplied so they can stabilize.[xiv]

As I walk away from my first meeting with NAMI, I realize maybe Daniel isn't as bad as the other sick people. After all, he hasn't been arrested and placed in jail. In hindsight, this is delusional thinking on my part because I didn't want to find myself in such a dire straight. I didn't want to admit our home is in chaos. I didn't want to allow mental illness to get a firm foothold in our lives. I don't go back because I rationalize things aren't so bad, that Daniel is okay, and his current medications will work longer with a better effect. I delude myself into thinking there will be no need for another hospitalization and I won't need NAMI.

Our family is growing as Tyler and Elizabeth have a beautiful baby girl named Ellen. She's such a treasure and so precious. It's important during a life mired in mental illness to stop and enjoy life's blessings as they occur. We're also really excited to see Karis finish her private university program and she graduates Magna Cum Laude.

Early in 2008, Daniel ends up back at our home because he's getting worse. Bob can't handle him in this state and he asks us to come and get him. One night, I awake to Daniel singing drunkenly at the top of his lungs in his bedroom. When I go check on him, he's completely wasted.

"Can I have the car keys?" I ask him, putting my hand out palm up. He readily hands them to me and I tell him to get some rest. When he's wasted like this it doesn't do any good to try and talk with him. He's belligerent and everyone else is the problem. He typically drinks over thirty-two cans of beer and then blacks out.

Another time, I wake to find Daniel at the side of my bed in the middle of the night… just standing over me, completely still, and staring. He isn't saying a word, just standing there. I know to remain calm and in control even though I'm startled and scared to find him there.

I force myself to act like this is no big deal and I'm not startled or afraid. "What's wrong?" I ask him.

"You need to take me inpatient. I'm sick." He responds in a flat, dead manner.

"No problem sweetheart, why don't you wait downstairs and I'll be right down after I change my clothes."

When I get downstairs and look into his eyes, I can tell he hasn't slept in a long time and his eyes are glassy and unfocused. We end up driving over to the crisis response unit in the early hours around 2 AM and ring their doorbell, hoping for assistance. On previous trips no one answered. This time they do and they tell us Daniel isn't sick enough for care, we have to go see our psychiatric care provider. We head home without help. I realize this isn't the way to get mental health care. To get aid, I need to take Daniel straight to the emergency room and have them call the crisis response unit after they check him out for a medical clearance. The medical clearance is to ensure there are no illegal drugs in his system which can cause him to be a danger to the staff. When Daniel is at our home, I know he can't find pills to take while he drinks alcohol as I keep all prescription drugs locked in our safe. He's known for stealing Bob's pain killers and mixing them with excess alcohol. It's important to figure out what a loved one is fixated on and to get that substance out of the home or locked up. I am starting to learn the system.

During 2008, Daniel slowly becomes more fragile and it's becoming obvious he's losing the fight for his health. Earlier in the year, Daniel left me a note saying, 'I'm going to die … Daniel' written in scribble. It has a chilling effect on me and I hope it isn't an omen. I know somewhere inside my son is a person with a gentle heart. Sometimes it good we don't know what lies ahead because if we knew, we wouldn't have the heart, strength, soul, or stamina to keep going.

# Part Two

# CHAPTER ELEVEN:

# Here We Go Again – March 2010

———————◆———————

*Without health life is not life; it is only a state of languor and suffering -*
*an image of death.*
*Buddha*

We've come full circle in March 2010 and are again trying to find a viable path forward. The past seven months were a bust in the mental health arena. Just as a reminder, Daniel was found outside his apartment nude, and we needed to intervene on his behalf before the manager called the police. My husband went to the apartment to pick him up and brought him out to our home. We're hopeful a bed can be found in a care facility as we know this situation is beyond our ability to manage. We get Daniel safely home and say a prayer of protection and provision for our son.

The next day, March 11, I head to Daniel's apartment in the early morning to clean up the beer cans and all of the garbage. I stop by the apartment manager's office to talk with him about Daniel's behavior.

"Daniel was nude outside his apartment numerous times over the last few weeks, and he was heard yelling profanities at all hours," he tells me. "The residents are becoming more and more disturbed by his behavior and they've made numerous complaints to me."

"Yesterday before I called your husband, I was on the grounds of the apartments working when I saw your son outside nude," he adds. "He was laying on the walkway outside his apartment up on his elbows sunbathing, his clothes lying at his side. I told Daniel to get his clothes on and he did what I asked."

I finish talking with the manager, which of course is very difficult, and I conceded there's no excuse for this kind of behavior. I feel guilty that I pushed Daniel onto the residents of this apartment. They have children to protect and everyone suffers. I leave the complex with only apologies for my son's behavior.

I head home because I hear Karen (Daniel's case manager) wants to talk to me and Daniel. I'm at a loss for what the next step looks like. Karen arrives at our home at 9 am and she asks Daniel, "Will you go voluntarily to the emergency room and then into the mental hospital? This will help us with a medication change because your behavior is getting increasingly erratic."

She turns to me and continues, "Unfortunately, the crisis response unit says there are no beds available today so you'll need to keep Daniel at your home."

"Let's proceed with a medication change today regardless of the bed situation," I tell Karen. "My husband and I will start the med change at our home today and hope a bed opens at the Grace Center tomorrow."

Later in the day Karen phones to say, "It's been determined not to start the medication change on an out-patient basis. We feel it will be best if he's in the hospital during this change." Karen is hopeful a bed will open tomorrow. "I'll get in touch with you in the morning regarding an available bed." Karen assures me.

Daniel's preoccupied with the voices all day and night. In the evening he asks me, "What's the worst crime?"

"Murder." I tell him.

A pause. "What about rape?" He asks.

I tell him they are probably equally as bad because they don't take into account the people they are gravely harming. A bit later I hear

142

him say in a fragment of his conversation with the voices, "Rape my mom," and "Cocaine." A minute or so later he tells me, "I'm a rapist."

I look at him and I tell him, "You aren't a rapist but a severely ill young man with a brain that's very sick and you need to stop listening to the voices. You've always been a kind, caring young man."

A couple minutes later, "Thank you, mom." He replies.

I sleep with the bedroom door locked and mace by my bedside. I start thinking I need to look into a guardian ad litem situation where under state law, a person is typically appointed for adult cases in which the individual is mentally ill or disabled. The guardian ad litem independently investigates the people they represent to determine if they're incompetent and which civil rights they can retain, such as the right to marry, to vote, to manage their own finances, and to live on their own.

I wake up early on the morning of March 12 and decide I need to write a letter to Grace Center, the clinic responsible for Daniel's mental health care, with the following people on distribution: Brian Pershall, MD.; Charles Egan, MD.; Sharon Watts, RN; and Karen Everett, Case Manager. The letter outlines my concern with the lack of mental health care and the pathway pursued by Dr. Egan. I know for a quick response I need to go in person to the Grace Center and ask that an original letter be placed in each of the four recipient's mailboxes.

The letter word for word in its entirety follows:

*March 12, 2010*

*Grace Center*
*Dr. Brian Pershall, Director*

*Brian Pershall, MD,*

*I'm compelled to write this letter in regards to the mental health care of our son Daniel Borders. Daniel has been struggling with mental illness since he was 14 years old, and he is now 28 years old. A great majority of the time has been with Grace Center under your excellent care. He spent a few years at New Hope under the care of Dr. Patterson. In August 2009 Daniel suffered a relapse where the meds he was on were unable to stop the voices. He went inpatient to Grace Mental Hospital at that time. It appears that today may be his 4th hospitalization since August 2009. He has deteriorated to the point that a least restrictive alternative agreement is needed, the voices are uncontrollable and leading Daniel in a gravely ill path. I'm greatly concerned at the lack of medicine that is being used in his care. There are numerous medicines that haven't been tried, and he was discharged in the beginning of January on only Abilify 2mg. We were told he would need to integrate the voices and learn to live with them. This is an unacceptable approach as the voices talk about murder, rape, killing me, and pornography. We don't want these voices integrated into Daniel, they need to be quieted. My concern is that after this 4th inpatient round he will again be released into the community as under medicated as the other 3 hospital stays. We were forced to move him out of our home for our own safety at the end of January 2010. In the 1 month he has been on his own he has continued to deteriorate further. He was arrested for being drunk in public & stealing beer and passing out outside of Right Drugs, and now appears to be on the road to a criminal record, which has never been the case during the previous 14 years. His medicine was raised to 5 mg Abilify 1 ½ weeks ago, and nothing else. Tuesday evening, he was found completely nude outside his apartment and yelling profanities, apparently this was not the first episode and the apartment tenants are very disturbed with his behavior. Leonard & I were phoned by his apartment complex to immediately intervene with Daniel. That same afternoon Leonard & I phoned Grace Center and spoke with his case manager in length about Daniel's bizarre behavior and our concern that he was under medicated. It could just as easily been the police arresting Daniel for the second time in 2 weeks. This lack of medication is ruining Daniel's ability to be in the community, process any logical thought and get well. I'm concerned for him, the community and our family. This letter is to outline my worry and to get your aid in ensuring that Daniel is adequately medicated so he can function in society and not be a danger.*

*Our family appreciates the care and concern of our team at Grace Center. But, something drastically needs to be changed regarding the approach being taken with Daniel. It is a dismal failure and Daniel and our family are paying the price.*

*I'm distributing this to his care givers, along with you, so that everyone knows my concerns and that as a team we can come up with a plan that is in Daniel's best interest and hopefully, his improvement with his schizophrenia.*

*Best regards,*

*Diane Borders*

*927-xxxx*

*Cc:*

*Charles Egan, MD*
*Sharon Watts, RN*
*Karen Everett, Case Manager*

After finishing the letter, I head to Grace Center and ask the receptionist to please place an original signed letter in each of the four recipients' mailboxes. She tells me she's happy to do this and takes my letters. I thank her and head home. Amazingly, later in the morning of March 12, Karen comes by our home and takes Daniel to Providence Medical Center for a medical clearance and the crisis response unit comes in for an assessment prior to his inpatient admittance to the Grace Center. I guess the letter had an effect. The director of the Grace Center is Daniel's old psychiatrist from age 16 to 21. I know Dr. Pershall will recognize the person

Daniel has become as not being the person he knew while he was under his care. My hope is that Dr. Pershall will step in and unblock the system so we can get Daniel care. It works and it looks like soon I'll be able to breathe again…at least for today.

This same morning, a Notice of Emergency Detention is filed with the Superior Court of the state. It is a petition for revocation of a 180-day LRA. James Livingston, Daniel's assigned lawyer, states the following:

*"The respondent will not take his prescribed medication. He is psychotic, responds to internal stimuli and talks about rage. He has no legal history and has been arrested for stealing beer. He admits to overdosing on medication. He cannot make a good faith decision for voluntary hospitalization. He would not be safe in a crisis respite due to non-compliance with medications."*

A treatment plan put together by Grace Center for this current stay lists the following issues: suicidal behavior, sexual preoccupation, delusional thinking, anger, and depression. These are important risk factors and issues they'll address during this hospitalization. From the intake paperwork, Daniel states he's using alcohol and cocaine. He's focusing on suicidal ideas and thinks that dying sounds good. He's spending a lot of time thinking about sexual scenarios and he thinks about raping girls, doing drugs, and drinking alcohol. In one minute he believes he's a Navy Seal and then a devil worshipper the next. He admits to using cocaine to try and overdose on purpose and is responding to hallucinations and making delusional statements regarding cultural issues. Dr. Egan orders Abilify for mood stabilization, Geodon for psychosis, and Melatonin for insomnia. Daniel is so psychotic he doesn't participate in any group activities.

I arrive at the hospital before visiting hours to bring clothes and Karen stops me outside the hospital to let me know Daniel tested

146

positive for cocaine on his hospital admission blood work. I am in shock. None of this makes any sense to me as we think the cocaine is just a delusion. Did things progress to the point where he acted out and found a way to sell himself for cocaine? Where did he get cocaine, he has no money?

Karen goes on, "Daniel told the doctor he's fantasizing about raping me too. The doctor doesn't want me anywhere near Daniel and they'll have someone else act as his case manager for my safety."

After we finish talking I'm left wondering how it's okay to have Daniel talking about doing the same thing to me and nothing is done for my safety, but when he says it against his case manager they are insuring he's nowhere near her.

When I get inside the hospital, I find he's being kept in isolation due to his sexual behavior. He's stripping nude and shouting profanities and is a danger to the other patients. He talks with Dr. Harvey, the inpatient psychiatrist, about raping his case manager and children in general. I'm not able to see Daniel because he's too sick. As I leave the hospital I phone Leonard telling him, "Don't come by because Daniel's too sick to be out with the general population."

Later in the evening, my husband and I discuss the strange results on his blood work and the cocaine in his system. "Is it possible we should've believed him when he told us he was using?" We determine I need to check with the nurses tomorrow at visiting hour to see what else his blood work might show.

I stop by the nurses' station on the second evening and ask, "Can I please get a copy of Daniel's drug test to keep in his file?"

As the nurse is looking it up to print out, she tells me, "The positive cocaine test is in fact an error and Daniel doesn't show illegal drug use at all."

I feel relief the illegal use of drugs isn't added to our list of issues to tackle. I'm glad this delusion is found to be just that, a delusion. However, we spent a fretful evening worrying about his future with extra stress. Even the medical staff at Grace is fooled into believing Daniel uses cocaine. I can't understand how we're told he used cocaine when the tests show he didn't, but I won't look a gift horse in the mouth; I'm elated Daniel isn't using drugs.

On March 15, I arrive to visit Daniel and bring him some clean clothes. A nurse grabs me when she sees me enter the ward and pulls me aside. She's been very helpful and concerned for Daniel. "We moved Daniel into an isolated room on a different wing from the normal rooms as he's acting out sexually and we don't want this affecting the other patients." She tells me. After a pause, she adds, "Daniel has schizophrenia."

I stand there speechless and feel an icy chill slide through my body. Time freezes and I can't concentrate or hear her anymore. It takes all the strength I possess to not burst out sobbing. My baby boy is now a schizophrenic and my world is shattered. I'm sure she has no idea I've never heard this label tied to my son before and she doesn't understand the import of her words. I hand her Daniel's clothing as soon as I can and ask her if I can leave by a side door which is near me. She takes out her key and lets me out of the locked psych ward.

I walk out of the door and stand in free, open space outside the facility. I'm rigid on the sidewalk leading to the parking lot and completely in shock. I feel light headed because I think I forgot to breathe. I wish my husband was with me to hold me and let me cry. I begin taking tentative steps towards my car and start crying for everything lost to us. I cry for the opportunities Daniel won't have and for the dreams we have to lay aside for our son's future. How did we come to this? How do I bear the pain of the loss of my son in every way that seems tangible? When I look at him now, there's no one home. He's lost in a delusion and I don't know if we can get him back from its grip.

I finally arrive at my car, get inside, and sit in muted silence, letting the situation wash over me as I try to come to terms with what this will mean to our lives. This diagnosis rocks my world and I can't figure out what I'm to do. I feel such anger wash over me at the lack of healing by God, and the anguish my son must face, how lonely his world must be…isolated and apart from everyone. I call Leonard and tell him what happened, crying softly and feeling helpless in the face of mental illness. I finally put the car in gear and head home not able to process this last hour.

The next day, Daniel has a mental health court hearing in the morning to discuss transferring him to the State Mental Hospital. We find out they'll move him when a bed opens at the state mental hospital. He's put on Geodon and Cogentin injections twice a day. We already know he was moved out of a normal room and put into isolation, but we find the staff is taping butcher paper over his window due to his sexual activities in the room. He acts out sexually and there are different bodily fluids spread through the room and the smell is overpowering. Women workers are no longer allowed into his room while he waits for his transfer to the state mental hospital.

The following morning, the state revokes Daniel's LRA and issues an order for his apprehension and detention. This is a formality because he's already in a locked facility. The state will detain him at the Grace Center and move him to the state mental hospital when a bed is available. James Livingston, MHP, files the facts of the allegations as follows:

*"Daniel is a 28-year-old male residing in Portland. He has a lengthy history of mental illness with multiple hospitalizations. He was placed on a 180 day LRA on 12-30-2009. The order was revoked on 3-12-2010 as the respondent had violated the terms and experienced a substantial deterioration in his condition. He admitted to having taken 2 weeks-worth of his medication over a period of 3 days in order to "lose weight". He was otherwise not taking his medication. He admittedly was consuming alcohol daily. He was observed by his case manager lying naked on his porch, "sunbathing". The respondent asked his mother whether "rape" was a horrible crime.*

*While at the Grace Center the respondent has remained sexually preoccupied. He has been observed by staff lying naked in his room with his door open and is visible to anyone walking by. His hygiene remains poor. He told staff that his favorite leisure activity is "raping girls". While he denies any hallucinations he appears to be internally preoccupied. His mood remains flat and he has considerable response latency. His ability to formulate ready responses is due to a lack of concentration caused by auditory hallucinations.*

*The respondent was interviewed for the purpose of a hearing and informed of his rights on March 17, 2010. He appears to be confused about the nature of the hearing.*

*The respondent acknowledged that he had been drinking, but could not or would not discuss his medication non-compliance. He demonstrated response latency and twice smiled inappropriately at questions. He was responding to internal stimuli which made it difficult for him to concentrate.*

*The respondent violated his LRA by consuming alcohol and not taking his medications as prescribed. It is the recommendation of the treatment team that his LRA be revoked to Grace Center and State Mental Hospital"*

*From Mr. Livingston's notes we learn Daniel admits to having taken two weeks' worth of his medication over a period of three days in order to lose weight.*

*On March 24, Leonard and I stop by and we leave Daniel a note because he's in isolation and is still not well enough to be in the general population. Leonard writes, "We stopped by to see you tonight but you were asleep. We love you and look forward to seeing you tomorrow, Love you, Dad & Mom." I add, "Love you Daniel."*

We're trying to help him remember his life before he reached this state, but I'm more afraid of him than before and I become apprehensive whenever we head out to see him. However, we're hopeful our presence will act as an anchor to reality and help him to try to get better.

When Leonard and I arrive to visit Daniel at the Grace Center the evening of March 25, we find out he was admitted to the state mental hospital on a revoked 180-day LRA. Daniel was transported via ambulance to the state hospital that morning and we weren't notified. Instead of being upset, we're both relieved he was transferred and we are hopeful they can do something for him.

The next morning, a state mental hospital case manager named Kelly calls to speak with Leonard and me to discuss Daniel. "Daniel's psychotic and he won't be released from the state mental hospital as long as the voices continue with their violent intent." Daniel is to be put on Risperdal, Effexor, and Lithium.

Kelly continues, "We see a huge problem with him drinking volumes and volumes of water or any liquid in a very short period of time. We're assigning 24-hour oversight, by way of a worker, to try to stop him from drinking fluids to such a copious level." This is the first time we know of this being an issue for him. This is definitely a new development.

On Monday, March 29, Daniel is assigned a new case manager named Tammy. She phones to let me know that on Thursday, April 1, there will be a conference call to come up with Daniel's seven-day treatment plan. She also tells me she isn't seeing Daniel exhibit any of the behavior that I described.

I ask her, "Can you speak to the Grace Center and let them tell you about his behavior in the community this last month, and his inpatient term prior to being transported to the state mental hospital?"

Tammy says, "I can't write a treatment plan based on his past behavior. I have to see it at the state mental hospital myself. He seems fine."

I am puzzled and wonder if his new medication change is working this quickly, especially since he's been on these medications before, they are nothing new in his treatment realm. Later in the afternoon, I check the legal website for court date appointments and find out Daniel has a court appearance scheduled for May 19, 2010. I contact the Grace Center and his psychiatric team at the state mental hospital to ask how to notify the courts he's inpatient at the state mental hospital. I phone Daniel's Indigent Defense Panel appointed attorney, Ellen Ridgley, to have her help me from the legal side of the court system on Daniel's behalf while he resides in the hospital because he will miss the upcoming criminal hearings. She's going to request an evaluation by the state mental hospital to see if Daniel is competent to stand trial. Daniel is charged with Theft 3, with a value of five hundred dollars or less.

## CHAPTER TWELVE:

# Keep My Son Hospitalized

———◆———

*Out of suffering have emerged the strongest souls; the most massive characters*
*are*
*seared with scars.*
*Khalil Gibran*

"On April 1st, Daniel will be present at a teleconference call, and we can all talk about his care and our plans for his release." This is the message left on my cell phone from Daniel's case manager at the state mental hospital. I'm shocked to hear they don't see anything wrong with him and they're going to release him. I spend some time talking with my friend and coworker, Jody, to get her advice on how to proceed from our family's point of view. I know this is my one shot to make an impact.

Jody tells me, "Have a list of the threats Daniel has made against you and ask him in front of the group if he still wants to do those things to you." I am preparing myself for the conference call knowing Daniel's life depends on them seeing the truth and keeping my son inpatient and receiving the mental health care he so desperately needs.

The morning of April 1, 2010, arrives and I enter my work office, shut the door, take a deep breath, and phone in to participate on the teleconference call. I whisper a prayer for the Lord to help know how to proceed. I don't want to act or respond in a way which is detrimental to Daniel. Sitting in on the call are Daniel's doctor, a case manager, an RN, a recreational therapist, a social worker, Daniel, and myself. His original admitting psychiatrist and original case manager are both away on vacation. I'm hoping the staff in attendance knows enough about Daniel to make this meeting productive. I already know Tammy, his current case manager, thinks he's well and ready for release from our telephone conversation a few days earlier.

I hear them talk about how Daniel is on a 'one-on-one oversight' due to his drinking huge volumes of water. They're concerned the Lithium he's taking is being flushed from his system before it can take effect. The hospital will request an Independent Living Skills evaluation and also a Chemical Dependency evaluation. During the course of their conversation I interject that Daniel's history shows him continuously drinking twenty to thirty plus cans of beer within one to two hours with the intent of blacking out and stopping the voices.

As the teleconference continues, I discover while at the hospital he's made inappropriate contact with females and they have to keep an eye on him to stop him from making unwanted advances. I can tell by their words they're going to release him and I begin to panic. I know my one chance is fast approaching to have my son show them his true thought patterns and intent, and help them see the ideas coming from the voices and delusions of which he's immersed.

I ask the team, "Can I talk to Daniel for a minute and ask him some questions?" The doctor says I can go ahead and then they wait and everyone goes quiet. I take a deep breath knowing this is my one chance to make an impact.

I ask, "Do you still want to rape me and others?"

He solidly answers, "Yes."

"Do you still want to sexually torture me?"

"Yes."

"Daniel, do you want to kill me?" I continue.

"Yes."

I ask, "Will you dismember my body after you kill me?"

He replies, "Yes." Forceful and without remorse.

"Are you a porn star?"

"Yes." He says clearly.

"Do you want to bludgeon blondes with a baseball bat?" My final question.

Without hesitation, he answers, "Yes."

You can hear a pin drop. I hold my breath and wait for their response. It's a very simple, straightforward exchange with no doubt as to the questions I asked and the answers he gave. I'm amazed these professionals didn't ask these questions of my son. I'm shocked they didn't look at the records from the Grace Center as a point of reference.

Finally, the doctor speaks, "We'll be increasing his medication and looking at the combinations being used for his psychiatric care. "The Abilify his doctor at home had him on should've been dosed at the 30 mg level, not 2 mg to 5 mg/day." In addition, the doctor states they'll transfer Daniel to the second or third floor ward when a bed opens up where it's quieter. These wings are used for long term care. The team also discusses that if Daniel is at their hospital longer than ninety days, his supplemental security income payment will be discontinued and the previous three months may be billed back to us. Also, the hospital team comments that we may want to consider temporarily relinquishing his apartment back home.

The doctor asks Daniel, "How would you respond if someone were to inappropriately approach you?"

"I'd let whatever happens, happen." He states this as if it's no big deal.

The team is silent again as they see the potential for the victimization of my son and those acts being welcomed by him. Not a normal response by any shape of the imagination. Many people suffering mental illness have hyper sexual desires where anything goes and is welcomed.[xv]

I ask the team about Daniel's criminal case in the District Court here in Multnomah County. I let them know his court case was moved from March 24th to May 19th. They say they'll send a letter to the court to let them know about my son's situation. They let me know a teleconference will occur again in three weeks at the one-month mark. We'll regroup at that point in time to see where we are with Daniel's care.

I hang up and take a breath. I didn't realize I had been holding it, waiting for the outcome. I can feel the adrenalin coursing through my body and I start to shake. I can't believe I've done it and my son spoke the threats out loud and in front of witnesses. I realize if he'd just sat there quietly and answered my questions denying the statements, he would've been released and these people wouldn't have a clue as to what they were releasing back into the community. I know Daniel will be there for at least a month and he'll get the care he needs from the staff at the state mental hospital.

Many people would look at this and think it strange for me to want to keep my son in the hospital, but I see it as keeping my son from victimization, not able to commit criminal acts, and to keep him alive. The relief is profound and yet my heart is heavy. My time is running out for finding a better approach to help him recover. The psychiatric medications only do so much; they obviously aren't stopping the hallucinations, voices, and delusions. I have to look for new ideas and accelerate my research while I still have the chance.

The next day we receive a written notice sent to Daniel for lease violation, informing us he needs to vacate the apartment. It isn't a shock. My husband and I will need to spend a weekend moving him out of the apartment and getting rid of his things. Even though he was only at the apartment less than two months, he burned holes in the new carpet and trashed the unit. We'll have to forfeit our deposit and offer to pay for all of the repairs to the unit. Our attempt to keep me safe from our son ended up in the destruction of an apartment. For the future, we'll know that isolating Daniel in his own apartment allowed the voices to take over and the delusions to win out. I'm not sure what a person is supposed to do in a situation like this when the system is no help and a life is in danger. At this point in time, I am assuming most families would have kicked their child out of the home, and they'd be on the streets homeless. I just can't do that. I have to try everything in my power to find an answer.

At the end of week one at the state mental hospital, Leonard and I make our first weekend visit. I'm filled with apprehension as we approach the hospital. This is the state mental hospital we heard about throughout our lives growing up in this region. I imagine the setting of One Flew Over the Cuckoo's Nest, as that is the only reference I have in my mind.

We take the back road to the hospital and drive past many old dilapidated buildings. My husband tells me they used one of the old buildings in the filming of a movie. He points it out as we drive by. It looks like a perfect setting to film a psychiatric horror flick because it has the feel of the old mental hospitals one would dream of in a nightmare. There's another old abandoned building and Leonard tells me this is where a riot broke out and hostages were taken. The story goes that the patients rioted to make a point about the horrible care they were receiving and the deplorable conditions they lived in, demanding to be treated like human beings. The inpatients riots ended peacefully and were found to be playing cards with their psychiatric team when the siege ended.

I tell my husband, "The patients must have wanted to spotlight the need for respect for human beings with mental issues." I didn't know Leonard was filled with so much knowledge about the history of this mental hospital. The building still stands and is surrounded by barbed wire. Leonard says it was an insane asylum for the violently mentally ill.

Our drive does nothing to alleviate my tension as I'm now thinking the worst about the facility our son is housed in. As we turn a corner, I see a beautiful lake beside the mental hospital. It's surrounded by trees and deer are everywhere. We find them lying by the entrance doors to many of the buildings, just sitting below windows on the grass in the shade. Just ahead of us we see a three story red brick building, much more modern than the ones we passed. It's a rectangular block with manicured grass and trees spotted throughout. Seeing the facility is a relief.

Leonard and I get out of the car and proceed to the receptionist desk at the very entrance of the building. We sign in at the front desk and they look through the items we're taking to Daniel. We have snacks we bought from the local farmer's market on the way to the hospital because we know Daniel might want to have some of his favorite foods. The receptionist reviews the hospital rules and conveys the visitation hours. The front desk staff are great and it feels like we're talking to normal, caring people.

We make our way through the hallways and outdoor corridors to an entrance of the hospital wing where our son is staying. We ride up in the elevator and get out on his floor and are met with a locked door and metal detectors. We push the button to summon help. One of the orderly's on Daniel's floor greets us and ushers us into a hallway where he tells us, "Put all of your belongings in one of these cubby holes. Take the key with you and you can retrieve your belongings when the visit is over." He checks through our bags again and lets us into the locked ward. He places my husband and me in the first room on the left and tell us, "Stay here and I'll bring you your son. It's not safe for you to wonder around so don't leave this area." We look at each other and settle in, anxious to see how Daniel looks and if he's improved any in the few days he's been at the hospital.

The orderly brings Daniel to us and we spend an hour visiting. Daniel shares with us, "They changed my medications to Risperdal 6 mg and Lithium 600 mg." He also says they stopped the Effexor because it was making him manic. He does pretty well the first half of our visit but then becomes preoccupied with the voices during the last half. He's laughing and talking with them as he looks over at people who aren't there. We can't tell what he's discussing as he's secretive with them and the conversation is in fractured whispers.

He proceeds to tell us, "I go outside and sit on a balcony for most of the day."

As Leonard and I are leaving, we are pensive and full of thoughts that are hard to process. We hold hands as we walk back to the main entrance.

"Is there really a balcony, and how would that work for the patients escaping?" I ask my husband. We're used to having delusions spun for us so we never know what's real and what is make believe. It's apparent the voices are definitely still in control and command all of his attention.

"I don't know, that doesn't make any sense," Leonard replies. We continue on to our car, both of us lost in our thoughts.

These same trips to the state mental hospital occur every weekend with many different scenarios playing out. Each visit leaves us wondering what's to come, how Daniel will look, will he be able to communicate or will he be absorbed in the voices? How long will he end up staying here? We never meet any of his psychiatric team during the nine months he's hospitalized, so all our communications are through telephone calls and voice messages. Meeting the medical caregivers and sharing insight with them is a pipe dream. There's no personal interaction with the doctor, case managers or staff. That's one of the good things about the local area hospital, you are able to meet the staff and interact to get feedback.

From visit to visit, Daniel tells us stories of events, upcoming discharge plans (which sends my adrenal system into overdrive with fear), medication trials, testing done, a brain MRI, blood draws for diabetes and thyroid, each played out for us in detail, and many times we wonder if they are based in reality. He tells us the staff tries many different drugs on him, they change them out and adjust the dosage as the month's pass. No positive results come out of any of the combinations of medications and we wait and hope for a change.

His depression lifts for a time, anxiety may be alleviated for a period of days, but the voices, delusions, and hallucinations remain. He doesn't seem to be aware of answers to basic questions and he's not grounded in reality. He's latent responsive (meaning he responds to our questions well after we ask the question) and we find him talking with his voices. He can keep it together for a short period of time, where if someone doesn't spend enough time with Daniel they won't see the psychosis. He's such a handsome young man and he's able to make people think he's well for a time. However, he just can't maintain the charade and it all falls apart. Most caregivers don't expend that much energy and time with an individual as their days are full with other clients. Luckily his case manager does invest the time and sees the behavior first hand.

Daniel's out of control when it comes to drinking fluids and he says it's to hydrate his skin. I look up the disorder which is tied to mental illness and fluid intake. It's called 'psychogenic polydipsia.' It's a type of polydipsia (excessive thirst) described in patients with mental illnesses and the developmentally disabled. It's present in a subset of people with schizophrenia. These patients, most often with a long history of illness, exhibit enlarged ventricles and shrunken cortex on their MRIs, making the physiological mechanism difficult to isolate from the psychogenic. It's a serious disorder and often leads to institutionalization as it can be very difficult to manage outside the inpatient setting. It should be taken very seriously as it can be life threatening because serum sodium is diluted to an extent that seizures and cardiac arrest can occur. Patients have been known to seek fluids from any source possible.[xvi]

Daniel has many changes to his psychiatric team over the months and I wonder how he copes with the constant shuffle of people in and out of his life. Being paranoid and delusional probably makes it hard for him to make connections of any meaning or to trust anyone.

On many of our visits he's quiet and doesn't talk much, then from out of nowhere he asks us, "How much of my beer did you throw out?" He lets us know he wants to go back to his apartment. I think his only concern is getting out and back to his alcohol consumption in the privacy of his apartment.

His case manager calls us to let us know, "After one month in the hospital, your son is still on one-on-one oversight on his newly assigned floor because of his excessive fluid intake and his inappropriate sexual behavior." He'll remain on the one-on-one for fluid oversight for seven weeks as they work to control the volumes of fluids he's drinking. Watching Daniel consume such huge quantities is amazing. Most of us would be throwing up if we tried to drink that excessively. When they stop the one-on-one oversight, Daniel is still out of control on his fluid intake but they can't afford to have one of their people tied up so long in trying to prevent him from drinking fluids. They resort to having blood draws which show them his health status and leave him to his own devices.

The case manager lets us know, "When we ask Daniel about murder or rape, he's forthcoming that he's in contact with Satan and takes direction from him. He's talking about raping the Johnson's baby." She asks us if we know anything about this line of thought.

We're not sure who or where that came from, as we know don't know any families by that name. We tell her, "We assume it's a delusion."

She continues, "He talks about raping people, especially anyone who resembles his old girlfriend, Barb. He sees nothing wrong with his thinking and he has no intention of discontinuing alcohol and sees no problem with its consumption."

One month into his hospital stay, Daniel says, "They wheeled me from my room that I share with Robert and put me into an isolation room." He vaguely remembers it happening. When he woke up around 3 AM, he remembered wrapping a sheet around himself because he was nude, and went out to ask the nurse why he'd been moved."

He says, "I was so groggy I don't remember her answer. The closet is small but I like it because I'm all alone." He smiles.

He's really disconnected and doesn't have the normal facial expressions or mannerisms you find in someone who is mentally well. We hear this information from our son but we haven't received any calls from the state mental hospital letting us know how things are going.

Daniel has a new case manager named Shawn, and he calls me to tell us, "Daniel's MRI results are back and they are negative." I feel disappointment in the MRI results because I was hoping for an easy out. A brain tumor is on my wish list, at least that way we have some reason behind this psychotic behavior. Shawn doesn't tell me anything else regarding the MRI test, and I really wish I had a copy of the doctor's interpretation of the MRI.

Shawn also lets us know, "Your son is now staying in isolation because his roommate is disturbed by him always stripping naked and aggressively humping the mattress and acting out sexually." This was the first time we heard from the staff that the story Daniel told us was true.

"He's still talking to the voices and is brutally honest about rape, killing, and still holds conversations with the devil. He shows no remorse or emotions to those around him, as if he's talking about the weather." Shawn is matter of fact about Daniel's symptoms and very calm. It helps me to hear him and learn. He continues, "Daniel says when he sees a person in the distance he fantasizes about raping them and how he would do it."

Ultimately, he's to remain sleeping in the isolation room for a total of nine weeks because he's talking about raping girls and is exhibiting aberrant sexual fantasies.

I speak with one of the caregivers about the sleeping arrangement and she says, "We don't have enough staff on the night shift to keep an eye on him, so he sleeps in the isolation room—which is really just a closet—at night to ensure everyone is safe."

Daniel's finally starting to acknowledge alcohol isn't healthy for him to drink and he needs to make some decisions about not drinking.

We receive a letter from the Department of Social and Health Services stating they're dropping Daniel from medical coverage because he's at the state hospital. They will reinstate his coverage when he's released from the hospital. This makes sense because he's no longer living in the community and he now resides in a confined hospital. I wonder what a person does if they don't have family to rely upon during times like these. If you are in the hospital and your supplemental security income stops coming in, how does a family keep paying rent for the ill person so they don't lose an apartment or a home? If the sick person is a parent, how do the children continue to eat while the sick patient is in the hospital? This must take a huge toll on the remaining family to fill in the gaps and take care of spouses and children left to fend for themselves. Daniel is fortunate he has us and we are fortunate he doesn't have a spouse or children to worry about.

During one of our visits, Daniel doesn't talk with the voices at all. He's extremely suicidal and depressed for the first thirty minutes of the visit.

I ask him, "Did you let the psychiatric team know how suicidal you are?"

"No," He replies, "and I won't take any medicine for this…I just want this to be over." He's angry and suffering. Thirty minutes later, the depression passes instantly and he spends the rest of the visit talking with us.

We let Daniel know, "If you are to ever live with us again the voices have to be controlled, and the content of the voices can no longer be taking over your thinking."

I interject firmly, "You can't drink alcohol, you have to take your medication, you have to go to bed each night, and you have to agree to Program of Assertive Community Treatment." We also discuss the care he's receiving at the state mental hospital and he agrees.

"I know I'm getting good help here and I need to stay."

Our visit was a roller coaster ride and I can imagine they're seeing the same shifting personality throughout the day. It's nice to see he recognizes he's getting good care at the hospital and he knows it's positive.

The case manager states on the phone during the week that Daniel may be at the hospital for a long time because the staff sees no improvement.

On one of our visits in mid-May, we let Daniel know, "We're moving your belongings back to our home and letting your apartment go."

He appears relaxed and we have interesting conversations on different topics. Daniel then tells us he visits with his Grandpa Claude every day. He says, "Grandpa talks about how much he loves me. We just talk about all kinds of random topics."

Leonard and I look at each other. Grandpa Claude (my father) has been dead since September 2000, almost ten years now. I'm not sure how I feel about this revelation. I know in life, Grandpa Claude and Daniel had a very close relationship. My dad felt an affinity towards him and during my dad's last three years, Daniel spent four to five days a week at my dad's assisted living apartment. Many nights he slept over and they'd talk about many different topics. Daniel loved his grandpa a lot and I know there's a huge void from his death. After he died, Daniel and I would sit for hours and talk about how much we missed him. I even spent most of the first three weeks wishing I could see my dad again just to hold him and let him know how much I missed him. One night in a dream, my dad came to me and told me goodbye and gave me a profound gift of knowing he resides in an awesome place and he's aware of all we're going through. This revelation helped heal the devastating sadness I felt at losing my dad. While he was alive, my dad knew all about Daniel's mental health issues and was heartbroken there wasn't any real help we were getting within our local community, or within the medical complex. When my husband and I left the facility and made our way back to our car, we wondered if the visits from my dad, and the conversations Daniel felt they had, brought him any peace. If they did, I was glad he had them. Any kind of peace in his life is welcome.

Since Daniel was admitted inpatient at the state mental hospital, we make sure he has some spending money in the form of one dollar bills so he can use the vending machines, and we also bring cigarettes and other snacks for him. He gets to smoke twice a day and they limit his cigarettes to two for each trip outside. He lives for the twice a day trips outside to smoke and he focuses his attention on that topic at every visit. We learn to time our arrival to be shortly after his smoke outing so he'll be less agitated and less focused on the time on the clock, wondering how many minutes left before they take the smoking group outside.

I'm following the status of Daniel's criminal charge online as this is the only way I get information on his case. I finally see he's charged with Criminal Non-Traffic. I'm not really sure what all of this means, but his charges are definitely real and will have an impact on any future apartments or jobs he might try to get.

As his court date rolls around, I phone the hospital and leave a message with Shawn, Daniel's case manager. "This is just a reminder of the upcoming court date. I'm assuming you've contacted the court system to let them know Daniel is up at the hospital. I'd hate to have him be a no show and have the court be unaware."

With relief, later that day I receive a phone call from Ms. Ellen Ridgley, Indigent Court Appointed Attorney, on our son's case. We talk about his illness, duration of sickness, and the gravity of his mental health situation and what we're experiencing on our weekly visits.

"I'll speak to the Prosecuting Attorney's Office about having the charges dropped as Daniel is gravely, mentally ill and not in possession of the ability to know right and wrong," she tells me.

Ms. Ridgley is a wonderful advocate for Daniel and our family; her assistance and insight is such a help in this stressful situation. It feels great to know we're in competent hands and she's looking out for Daniel's best interest and knows how to work the legal system. This is an area our family has no experience with and I know I can call her if I need to talk about the case.

Ms. Ridgley states, "Daniel didn't drink any of the beer he stole. He stopped right outside of Right Drugs, sat on the ground, and passed out because he was already drunk when he stole the beer. The police found him there, he handed them the beer, and was compliant and cooperative as they took him to jail. The jail notified the mental health system to come and get him the next morning because he was obviously mentally ill." It's nice to hear how the incident went down in more detail. Ms. Ridgley lets me know Daniel's next appointed court date is June 30.

In late May on a visit, Daniel is still talking about the same topics and showing no remorse or regret about his violent sexual thinking and ideations. When we're with him this visit he appears relaxed and conversational.

Daniel wants to arm wrestle me. I look over at my husband who is smiling. I say, "Sure, but I'm not very strong." We arm wrestle, and I beat him without trying at all. I thought he was being funny by not trying, but he seriously thought he tried. It surprises him to see how weak he has become. We encourage him to use the exercise time and the weight room during his sessions to strengthen his muscles. The hospital has exercise periods and maybe now that he recognizes his lack of muscle strength he'll make use of the opportunity. He was already weak and nutrient deficient before this last psychotic episode and being in a hospital setting can't help. We hope he remembers and imagines it helpful...maybe he'll try.

At a later visit, a nurse named Vickie tells me they're talking about trying Zyprexa or Haldol as options for Daniel's medications. She lets me know he says he won't take Zyprexa. She is surprised he's so against the medication.

"He has some experience with Zyprexa and that may be why he doesn't want to try it again," I tell Vickie. "He probably isn't open to the Zyprexa as it really made him gain weight when he tried it years ago. At that time, he put on fifty pounds and started getting stretch marks in his skin so we stopped the medication. He hasn't tried Haldol, so maybe that'll be a good one to try." Maybe it holds the key to his recovery.

I notice Daniel appears to have gained ten pounds quickly from when we saw him two weeks before. He says, "I drank three gallons of water since yesterday afternoon trying to flush the toxins out of my system." He believes it's to help get the alcohol cleaned out.

Vickie speaks with him about the importance of just drinking a cup of water every hour and to control his intake so he can get better. He seems open to that thinking but I doubt he'll follow through.

"Do you know anything about my court case?" He asks.

He's wondering if I know anything about the charges. I go over everything I learned from his attorney and after we were done talking, he changes the subject. Daniel is still talking about his delusions of cocaine use and how he's now stopped taking cocaine. He doesn't realize yet that this is a delusion. He doesn't realize he never took cocaine and always tested clean. This is one visit that was all over the map, but at least he's communicating. His mind is a jumble of thoughts.

By mid-June, Daniel tells us he's now sleeping in a room with Robert instead of in the isolation closet at night. This must mean they have seen some kinds of positive change in his behavior.

In late June, Leonard receives a call from a woman named Sage at the state mental hospital. Sage tells him, "Daniel's LRA expired in early to mid-June. I'm at the hospital to evaluate Daniel and I find him stable and ready for release."

Leonard responds with, "Woo…Who are you and why am I not talking to Daniel's caregivers?"

"I'm the person sent to evaluate Daniel for a potential least restrictive alternative agreement and I find him stable," she responds with authority. "Because he's stable, I won't issue a new LRA." I immediately phone Daniel's case manager, Shawn, upon hearing the news from Leonard to find out what in the world is going on with the LRA. In the room on the conference call are Daniel's doctor, Shawn, a designated mental health professional, and my son.

Shawn confirms, "We received a hot call today to alert us that Daniel's LRA has administratively fallen through the cracks and we no longer have the protection of being able to detain Daniel against his will when he's released from the hospital if he doesn't comply. Due to this error, legal power to intervene is now gone. Daniel can only stay at the hospital if he volunteers to stay."

To say I'm pissed off is an understatement. "I worked so hard in this state mandated system to get my son care and force the system to pay attention to all of the disorder in his life, now I hear your mistake makes it possible for him to walk out the hospital."

"Daniel volunteered to stay." They tell me.

Shawn picks up from there, "But because of the error, when Daniel is released he won't be under a LRA when he's out in the community. We'll no longer be able to force compliance with his medications, keeping his appointments, and not drinking alcohol."

I sit stunned and at a loss for words. Daniel speaks up, "I'm not thinking of murder, rape, or torture and I haven't for the last three weeks."

I ask him, "Are Satan and Loci still with you, giving you direction?"

"No, they're not." He responds. In the past Daniel said Satan and Loci are where he gets all his power, and Loci gives him directions. He believes all the good things happening to him in his life are from Satan. I want to know if these entities are still front and center in his psyche.

The case manager asks me if Daniel can return to our home. "We have been through hell since November 2009. I have to know Satan and Loci are gone, and Daniel is truly well." I respond. I also let them know our home is one hundred feet from a public access walkway around a lake; and Daniel will be without supervision from 6:30 AM to 5:00 PM Monday through Friday while Leonard and I are at work.

"Do you know for sure Daniel's safe in the public where anywhere from ten to twenty children walk, ride bikes, and fish right at the end of our back yard?" I ask emphatically. "If you release him out into the community without housing planned beforehand, you're responsible for anything bad that happens to innocent people outside our home and in the community." I bluntly state.

I also let them know I'm keeping a log of every event, every person I am dealing with, dates, times, medication changes, attempts at getting care, being turned away from a crisis bed during psychotic episodes, and every lapse in care that occurs. I want the state mental hospital on notice that this entire saga is being tracked and listed out in case we need this information down the road. I'm so furious I can hardly think straight.

When I hang up the phone, I feel completely let down by these systems. I immediately call my husband, "Do I have to do my job and their job at the same time? Do I have to watch all of their deadlines too? Do they not have any professional responsibility to perform their jobs and not let our most important least restrictive alternative agreement fall through the cracks?" I'm beside myself with worry now that I don't have the protection of the LRA. We'll have to wait for Daniel to get terribly sick again, after he's released from the state mental hospital, in order to get another one instituted.

When I get home from work in the evening I dig through my official paperwork to find the most recent LRA. At 9:30 in the evening, I phone Shawn and leave a message at his work telling him

I have the agreement in my hands which has signatures for a six month LRA that is dated December 30, 2009. Won't this make his current one good until June 30, 2010? Don't we have eight more days to get the correct papers enforced?

The next morning, Shawn phones me to let me know he immediately contacted the lady who is in contact with the County Court to confirm the LRA was initiated on December 14, 2009, even though all signatures and the court hearing were on December 30, 2009. Apparently, even though all five documents were completed and signed on December 30, 2009, the clock started ticking on December 14, 2009.

"From a legal standpoint that sounds incorrect. The signatures are what make the contract valid, and they were signed and noted on the 30th." I tell Shawn. I think it's criminal the LRA is allowed to expire, especially after all the trauma our family has gone through since last summer."

"How long does voluntary mean?" I ask him.

"Daniel will be at the state hospital until he's discharged as stable."

"What's the definition of stable? Sage found our son stable yesterday and only one week earlier he'd finally been allowed to sleep in his own room instead of in isolation because of his sexual promiscuity, and he's still drinking huge amounts of fluids, so what constitutes stable?" I ask.

"If Daniel begins to decompensate, we'll hold him and contact the crisis unit in Salem to come and do an evaluation." Shawn replies.

"Daniel won't be allowed to return to our home." I respond, though it breaks my heart.

Shawn agrees, "I completely understand."

Daniel needs a controlled environment in order to get and stay well and I believe a group home may give him that control. I float the idea by Shawn. "Leonard and I won't always be around and we need to find a suitable group setting where Daniel will be happy, settled, and cared for as he ages." Now that I've started, I can't seem to stop. "If he's released on his own into society, he'll immediately drink alcohol by any means necessary and we'll begin the cycle again, like we've done for the last eight years."

I am exhausted and in my mind I'm running through this whole scenario again. While Daniel was in his apartment, his weight went down to 137 pounds because he didn't concern himself with food, only alcohol. Multiple times Daniel threw away his medicine because he believed he was well. A controlled environment is mandatory for his improvement and well-being. Every time he decompensates we're back with the fixations of murder, rape, sexual torture, Satan, and Loci. It's a never ending loop because he only cares about alcohol and his medications don't stop the voices, delusions, and hallucinations. No matter his words, his actions don't match. Then the horrific voices and their influences start again. I am at a loss and feel hopeless.

Shawn continues our discussion, "When the hospital determines Daniel is stable and we release him, we plan on having a chemical dependency assessment. He'll probably be inpatient in the state somewhere. When he's discharged, he'll be forced onto the Program of Assertive Community Treatment, which is a small, intensified program where a specialized team will check in on him daily to ensure medication compliance."

"When you discharge him, can our son can be sent to a 24-hour care home?" I am trying not to sound like I'm begging.

"We can't force him to choose a 24-hour care facility." Shawn answers.

A week later, Leonard and I go to visit Daniel in the afternoon. I am nervous I'll find our son asking to be discharged and wanting to go back home since he's here on a voluntary basis now. I'm praying God will keep my son locked up until he's well enough to be in the community.

The nurse greets us. "I'm glad to see you brought him beef jerky, he really needs to increase his salt intake. We're extremely concerned about his electrolytes due to the massive amount of fluids he drinks each day, but we don't have the staff to monitor him. He could die easily with the situation the way it is. We're monitoring him through blood work to keep an eye on his electrolytes and fluid status. Your son is categorized as Categorically Needy." I'm incredulous. If Daniel is this ill, how come they don't see a need for a least restrictive agreement?

In late June, I call and talk with Ms. Ridgley, Daniel's attorney, because he's due in court the next day. I phone in the morning and tell her, "Daniel's still up at the state mental hospital and can't make his court appearance on June 30, 2010."

"A warrant will not be issued for his arrest." She replies.

She also adds that three weeks ago, an evaluation order was sent to the state mental hospital for them to complete. She's expecting to receive a response that the hospital will determine at the time of the crime Daniel didn't have the mental capacity to show intent. The next day, she calls back to tell us a warrant won't be issued.

During the nine-month hospitalization, I hear from Daniel many times that the staff at the hospital are working on his discharge papers. Every time it churns my stomach and I make calls during the following days to see if this is correct. So far, none of the stories are true.

In many of my talks with Daniel's case manager, I let him know I don't want Daniel to return to the doctor we had in our local community due to his lack of medication knowledge and how desperately ill he became under this doctor's care. Shawn says he'll make a note of that on Daniel's charts for when discharge appears imminent.

At one point during the hospital stay, I contact Shawn to tell him, "Our other son Tyler had a blood test showing he has a genetic mutation MTHFR A1298C and I was wondering if you could test Daniel for the same abnormality." MTHFR is a genetic mutation tied to the methylation pathway which I've been reading about for many years, primarily from Dr. Yasko. I'm surprised to see Tyler actually has one of the mutations in his blood work.

"Do you think if Daniel has this mutation it could affect his mental state especially because of his alcoholism and how it impacts the nutrient levels in the body?" I ask. The hospital declines to answer my question, dig deeper into this issue, or test for the gene mutation. This is something I'll need to do in the future after Daniel is released, and when he is well enough to comply.

In late July when Leonard and I visit with Daniel, he's quiet. I'm shocked to see him smirking, smiling, and silently laughing as we wind down the visit. It's obvious he's still internally preoccupied with the voices. This surprises me because it's been less obvious the past few weeks. I hope the psychiatric team sees what we see.

At the same time, the state mental hospital completes and delivers their forensic evaluation of Daniel for the county court system to help determine if he's well enough to stand trial for his crime.

Daniel was evaluated by Mr. Tony Frolen, Ph.D. Mr. Frolen's notes state:

*"Mr. Borders was admitted to SMH on March 25, 2010, on a revoked 180-day LRA from Multnomah County:*

*He initially focused on his alcoholism, which he has used for an extended period. With specific questioning, he also endorsed multiple other symptoms, as he stated that he has bipolar disorder and schizophrenia. Apparently, Mr. Borders had been off his medications and was drinking heavily.*

*Mr. Borders has had been multiple hospitalizations and has gone to Detox three times and the MICA program twice. He stated that he did not stay because he did not like the program. At the time of his admission, Mr. Borders was taking Geodon, thiamine and melatonin.*

*According to the mental status examination, Mr. Borders was exhibiting obvious internal preoccupation. In addition, he stated that he has very violent thoughts that he will hurt someone or rape someone. Mr. Borders is clearly psychotic.*

*On July 8, 2010, Mr. Borders was 103 days into his hospitalization. He was prescribed Risperdal and Lithium. Although he appeared to be making slow progress, it was still clear that he has not fully recovered from his psychotic break. He continues to reside at the state mental hospital at the time of this letter.*

*It is my opinion that Mr. Borders continues to suffer from a mental disease or defect—schizoaffective disorder—and because of symptoms associated with this mental disease or defect, he continues to lack the capacity to assist in his own defense.*

*It is my recommendation that the court considers dropping the charge and allows Mr. Borders to continue receiving treatment on the Adult Psychiatric Unit at SMH.*

*It is my opinion that if Mr. Borders stops taking his medications again and/or starts drinking to excess again, he would be a substantial danger to other persons and would present a substantial likelihood of committing criminal acts jeopardizing public safety or security, unless kept under further control by the court and or other persons.*

*According to his NCIC, Mr. Borders has no felony or misdemeanor convictions.*

*As stated in the mental status exam during admission, Mr. Borders endorses violent thoughts that he would hurt someone or rape someone when he is not taking his medications. Adding alcohol to this mind set significantly increases the risk for recidivistic antisocial behavior of a potentially violent nature."*

The following day a copy of Daniel's evaluation is faxed to the county court judge with the hopes the court will drop the Third Degree Theft charge against Daniel due to his mental illness. I'm holding my breath while we go through this process. I hate to see my son with a criminal record and I hope to keep his record clean and free from criminal charges. We work so hard to keep him safe against all obstacles.

In early August I contact Ms. Ridgley to ask, "Did you receive the court mental evaluation document from the state mental hospital?"

"Yes I have, and I believe the court charge will be dropped." I let out a sigh of relief. Finally, something good. "I'll let you know what happens at the hearing tomorrow." She adds.

The same day we find out Daniel's old grade school friend, Dena, wrote him a letter letting him know he's in her thoughts and she hopes he makes a recovery soon. It's so nice to know that a person from his past still thinks of him and wishes him well, and encourages him when it seems so hard to find any kindness shown his way.

I feel a huge burden lifted off my shoulders when we're informed that state Court Case Number M000xxxxx against our son is closed. I send up a silent prayer thanking God that he was with us during this time and was able to influence people on our behalf, and choreograph circumstances. Our son doesn't have to go to jail. I've known people who have mentally ill loved ones in hospitals that upon release are required to complete jail time for crimes committed while they were mentally ill. Ultimately, we can shut the book on this horrible arrest.

In August I receive a copy of the Department of Social and Health Services Competency, Diagnosis, and Opinion regarding Daniel's status. The information clearly states if Daniel stops his medications again and/or starts drinking, there's a substantial likelihood of his committing criminal acts and jeopardizing the public safety or security unless kept under further control by the court or other persons. It also endorses Daniel has violent thoughts and he may hurt or rape someone when he's not taking his medications. Adding alcohol to this mindset significantly increases the risk for recidivistic antisocial behavior of a potentially violent nature. As I read this, I'm amazed the LRA has been allowed to expire and the state mental hospital doesn't see the need for a new LRA to be instituted.

On August 4, our daughter Karis returns from a year of legal aid volunteer work in Minnesota. I've missed her so much and am happy to have her home. She had her share of growth events and hard times during the last year. We spent many phone calls visiting as she worked her way through the year. She saw such heartache in the community and so many situations seemed futile. A few of the clients from restraining order court were murdered during the year and it was emotionally draining for her. I hope she has time now to chill and recharge herself.

Daniel spends his birthday in the mental hospital. We ask him, "Can we bring you something special for your big day?"

He says, "I'd like a cherry pie." We tell him we'll bring one with us to celebrate his birthday when we return.

When Karis hears about the request she immediately wants to bake the pie. She's looking forward to seeing him on his birthday. I believe the greater value put on things, the more care goes into their recovery. Our children are everything to us; and I know a day is coming when my son is going to be released from the state mental hospital while he's still quite ill.

In preparation of this, Karis and I start a twelve-week program through the NAMI called Family-to-Family. The class is for families of people with mental illness. The goal is to teach us about mental illness, equip us with tools to help us deal with stressful situations, and keep ourselves well too. The class is very helpful and it's good to share our stories of pain with other families who can relate. The NAMI training focuses on teaching us how to be part of the psychiatric team for our mentally ill loved ones.

The first day of class as I look through the curriculum, I see a session on communication and I know this is a day I'm going to skip. I look over at Karis and say, "This is a class I don't need; let's skip it." She agrees and we decide on the communication night we'll go out for pizza instead.

I tell Karis, "I've been communicating with Daniel for seventeen years; I think I know how to talk to him. I mean he's still alive."

But then a funny thing happens. Karis and I skip the communications class only to find out at the next session the topic for the night is communication. I look over at Karis and smile. "There must be a reason why we need to be in this class tonight."

We perform a role-playing exercise where some people in the class are assigned the role of a schizophrenic and the others are assigned the role of their voices. Karis is one of the schizophrenics and I'm one of four people who will stand behind her and read the same statement over and over. The four of us have different statements to read at the same time. While we each read our individual cards out loud, Karis tries to follow the most elementary directions by the teacher. She is to perform the task on paper as the teacher gives her direction. Karis tries to hear the directions as the four of us are talking behind her. She finds it almost impossible and is greatly impacted by the knowledge that Daniel lives with this scenario all day, every day, and all the while we're expecting him to perform normally.

I learn I'm communicating all wrong with Daniel. While I think I'm doing a great thing by not responding in fear and by hiding my thoughts, I find out that in truth, Daniel could care less about my thoughts and feelings. He's so wrapped up in his own illness and delusions that I am irrelevant in the grand scheme of things.

I am making myself sick by hiding all of my thoughts and emotions. I need to tell Daniel what I'm thinking at the time each episode occurs. I always assumed if I told him my thoughts and feelings it would cause him to commit suicide and it would be on my shoulders for the rest of my life. It's a relief to hear it's okay to verbalize my thoughts. This will come into play when they release Daniel from the state hospital because I know he'll somehow end up back with us because the system will fail us again.

At the NAMI Family-to-Family class we meet many families just like ours struggling with mental illness and all of the stories are heartbreaking. People from all walks of life, religion, and social status attend these sessions. No one is immune. Every time I try to tell a part of our story, I find myself in tears as the pain is too great to speak out loud. I'm devoid of hope and am very angry at God for the lack of healing for my son. I don't want any more prayers said for him and I tell my husband not to pray anymore in front of me for Daniel's healing. I know God isn't deaf, so if healing isn't happening, I must find the answer to what I'm supposed to be doing.

On Daniel's 29th birthday, Karis brings him a cherry pie, as promised, and gingerbread boy cookies because she knows these are also his favorites. Daniel's quiet today and not very talkative, however, he tells us, "I get out in early September. I had a talk with the case manager four or five days ago."

He continues, "I'll be staying at the Connor House in Portland, and I chose the Program of Assertive Community Treatment as my caregivers when they release me."

I wonder if he chose PACT because of the talks we had earlier. This team will make his care more stable and help with his overall support.

"I like the idea they'll come to me and I won't have to worry about how to get to my appointments and refill medications." He tells us. I hope he keeps thinking positively about PACT because they'll be so helpful in managing his medication compliance. Especially now that we don't have a LRA in place.

"I started Haldol 5mg and I'm feeling less angry and I'm having less violent thoughts." Daniel lets me know. "Before the new drug, I was walking around feeling really angry, and I feel like the medicine is helping."

"I'm hopeful Haldol will continue to make you feel even better as the medicine builds up in your system." I respond. "It's encouraging that you're feeling less anger. It'll be nice to see even more positive changes that make you feel even better." This is a drug we haven't tried before so I'm crossing my fingers and praying for success. I realize I sound confused as I ask for no more prayers for Daniel, and yet in my quiet space I am still praying for each and every outcome on every situation we face. I am very disconnected emotionally, yet vulnerable and needing somehow to find peace.

I learn through a phone call a couple days later the hospital isn't considering placing him in a group home yet because they believe they can get him better first, so no release is forthcoming. Each time he tells me that he's being released, I feel fear well up inside. I need to learn to cope with this because it'll happen eventually, so I better start getting ready.

While on the call, Shawn tells me, "Daniel's still responding to outer stimulus but denies it. Daniel says he hasn't had thought of murder, rape, or sexual torture for the last couple months."

A week later, in early September when Leonard and I visit with Daniel, we bring hair clippers with us and my husband ask the staff, "Can my wife cut Daniel's hair because it's getting so long?" They're happy to allow me to cut Daniel's hair and they take us to a room that has a vinyl floor where we can clean up afterwards. Daniel's hygiene is so bad that I have to ask him to shower first because his hair is packed tight with dried conditioner he doesn't wash out. He thinks if he leaves the conditioner packed in his hair it'll cause his hair to turn blonde and he likes the idea of being blonde.

The results of the shower aren't great because the product is pretty caked on, and one washing isn't enough, but I cut his hair anyway. It's nice to be doing such a routine thing with Daniel and it feels normal. If I can just change the surrounding I can make believe he's young again and at home getting his hair trimmed.

When I'm done, his hair looks great and he seems happy with the results. I hope by doing something as mundane as cutting his hair, it might give him a bridge back to remembering normalcy. He's more talkative today, but while I'm cutting his hair he's whispering to his people and carrying on a conversation with them. I can't make out what he's saying because it is covert, but it's there.

# CHAPTER THIRTEEN:

## Keep My Son Sheltered

———◆———

*Health is the soul that animates all the enjoyments of life, which fade and are*
*tasteless without it.*
*Lucius Annaeus Seneca*

In late September Leonard, Karis, and I arrive for a visit with Daniel. He's more talkative this weekend than the one before. During the visit, he begins laughing really hard as he says, "I stole beer from the same Right Drugs store four different times." This is the same Right Drug where he was arrested. He thinks this is hilarious and I realize we really have our work cut out for us. I don't see much improvement in his psychosis. This tumultuous road has a long way to go and I know I need to be searching diligently for an answer to this mental illness, and quickly, because our time is running short.

In mid-October Leonard visits Daniel alone because I have a cold and he brings a photo album of Daniel from birth through middle school. They look through the pictures during the visit and Daniel asks, "Can I live with you and mom when they release me?" Leonard remains silent for a moment trying to figure out how to respond and Daniel then asks, "Or can I have my own apartment?" Eventually he tells Daniel yes to both questions.

That evening Leonard is recounting his conversation to me and I tell him, "Daniel can't stay with us."

"I know, but I just can't say the words out loud." He's struggling with the feeling of letting Daniel down, and hurting our son. He can't imagine how this situation is going to go down when the state

185

releases Daniel from the hospital because neither of us are seeing enough improvement to warrant his release.

"We already tried the apartment and it was a huge catastrophe, and it made Daniel worse." I remind him. "With him fixated on hurting me, I'm not safe alone with Daniel either. I'm not sure what we should do, but we don't have any safe options when the hospital lets him out."

Leonard can't bring himself to say 'no' and hurt Daniel. He tells me, "We don't know when he'll get out of the hospital, so let's not worry until then because it could be a long way off as sick as he is right now."

One weekend later when we visit, Daniel is laughing and tells us, "I drank at least twenty cups of coffee. I put ice in to chill it so I could drink it faster. When it's hot, I have to sip it and I can't drink as fast."

I can't even imagine drinking that much of any beverage quickly and why anyone would want to do it in the first place. Leonard and I are looking at each other sitting here in the room with Daniel wondering when we'll start seeing the medication changes kicking in.

"Because I drank so much it made me run to the toilet to throw up, but I didn't make it and I threw up outside the bathroom on the floor," he continues. He's laughing as if it the funniest story he's told us yet. "No one saw me, and I didn't tell anyone about the mess I made. It just looked like someone spilled a pot of coffee filled with coffee grounds." He's laughing about it, thinking it's hilarious.

I ask him, "Was that the first time your vomit looked like coffee grounds?" I am worrying about why his vomit would have that consistency and did we need to worry about bleeding going on in his gastrointestinal tract?

While I'm still thinking through this piece of information, his dad let's him know, "You need to let people know when you throw up so they can clean up the mess so others won't walk through your body fluids." Daniel just continues laughing again at the hilarity of the situation.

He's also laughing when he changes the subject with, "My roommate Dustin gives me chew. Dustin chews and spits, but I chew and swallow." Just the thought of it makes my stomach roll.

He continues, "When I go out on smoke breaks, I throw up outside."

"Does anyone see you?" I ask, hoping this is a delusion, but sensing it may be true.

"No," he replies, "I stay off in the corner by myself so no one sees it happen."

The inpatient group is led outside by an orderly who lights their cigarettes and keeps an eye on the group. He often tells us that Daniel stays apart from the group and hasn't made any friends so I can see this happening. "The chew helps me make it to the next smoke break." Daniel says.

I ask him, "Why are you swallowing when you should spit it out?" I can't imagine purposefully swallowing chew.

"To lose weight." He responds. He's 150 pounds now. After having lost fourteen pounds, he wants to be thinner. I try to talk to him about the extreme health risks he's taking and he just laughs and doesn't seem to have any idea of the consequences of his behaviors.

The topics change randomly and Daniel says, "I don't communicate with anyone at the hospital; I just stay to myself."

"You should make an effort to get to know the people here because maybe they can help you feel better if you talk to them." Leonard replies.

Without responding, Daniel starts on a new topic, "I haven't seen my case manager since the first month I was brought up to the second floor; I see my doctor only once a month." I'd be surprised if this statement is true because Shawn talks about his meetings with Daniel and how his Activities of Daily Living assessments aren't good.

The following Monday, I let Daniel's case manager know about the vomiting of coffee outside the bathroom so they are aware of what he's doing. In late October Daniel tells us they're monitoring his coffee intake and will only allow him three coffees. He's a handful to monitor because he won't change his behaviors due to how his mind works.

He then moves quickly on to, "I met with a lady to discuss my release plan. I want to live with you guys." My heart falls at the notion they think he's well enough to discharge.

I tell Daniel, "You'll need to complete a 90-day stay at the Connor House to ensure you're stable enough in the community first."

Daniel shifts gears rapidly again and says, "I'm still chewing and swallowing because I like how it makes me feel when I swallow. I know I shouldn't drink because it makes me not well," he interjects. The topics are changing swiftly, so we just sit back and listen. Each of us in our own world, trying to process the information, wondering if it's true or not and how to respond.

Knowing I've said this before, I tell him, "Alcohol makes your brain really sick and if you don't drink you can be successful in whatever you choose to do." I'm trying to give him hope. I used to think if we could stop the alcoholism, maybe his mind would be retrievable, but now I realize he's been in the hospital since March, alcohol free, and we still don't see any improvement. It's a pretty sad and sobering realization. The entire visit leaves me reeling with questions, worries, and fear of the future. Daniel isn't well and our time is running out.

# CHAPTER FOURTEEN:

# Keep My Son from Hurting Us

———————◆———————

*We consume our tomorrows fretting about our yesterdays.*
*Persius*

On November 1, 2010, Daniel's case manager Shawn calls to tell me the state mental hospital is going to release Daniel on November 2. I'm stunned into silence while he lays out the plans. The day I've been dreading is here.

Shawn continues, "The hospital will drive Daniel in a van to Connor House in Portland where he's approved for up to three months. There will be no LRA in effect as the document expired, so we'll have no power to make him conform to certain guidelines. Karen Everett will again be his case manager through the Grace Center."

My mind goes back to the error they made in letting the LRA expire, and not replacing it with a new one because they didn't think he needed it anymore.

I let Shawn know, "I worry Dr. Egan will again be Daniel's psychiatric doctor and he had Daniel on virtually no medication. I can't imagine him in charge of my son's care again." My mind goes back to our past experience with Daniel not taking his medication, and how I can't imagine anything's changed, so I continue by asking Shawn, "Will Daniel be in the PACT program? He'll need someone to help him comply with appointments and medication compliance."

The PACT program assigns special assistance and caregivers who ensure Daniel's daily medications, life needs, alcohol consumption, etc. are all monitored. They make sure he's successfully taking his needed medication. Since this isn't in place, the odds of him complying with his medication and alcohol needs are slim to none, as he doesn't believe he's ill.

After interviewing Daniel in the state mental hospital, the forensic psychiatrist wrote if Daniel were to be off of his medication and/or drink alcohol, he could become a danger to the community. Without the LRA, this scenario is likely to play out.

Shawn responds, "I'll phone Karen and let her know the state mental hospital doesn't want Daniel's medication messed with by Dr. Egan." This gives me a little bit of relief. Shawn can't confirm Daniel will be in PACT. "Karen will have to work the topic when Daniel gets home." I'm already seeing the writing on the wall. His release isn't positioned for success.

Immediately after I hang up with Shawn, I phone Karen regarding Daniel's upcoming release. She confirms no LRA is in effect as it fell through the cracks up at the state mental hospital, and the paperwork wasn't completed in time. I knew this from the fight I had with the state mental hospital at the time they let the LRA lapse. This was the first Karen knew of the state hospitals lapse in paperwork. She is apprehensive, but feels it's just a matter of waiting for Daniel to decompensate so he can be detained again, at which time he'll return to the Grace Center and we can get another LRA in effect again.

We have two choices in our area for housing for Daniel. One is the Connor House and the other is the Elijah House. "The Connor House is willing to give Daniel a chance," Karen tells me. "The house manager knows about Daniel's past. The manager also said the mental health workers at the home are all young, inexperienced, female staff, and they're green." I hope they're able to deal with my son.

"The Connor House has zero tolerance for alcohol and Daniel will be kicked out if he drinks. If they do kick him out, I feel it best if we let him be homeless on the streets as he made the choice to drink." Karen believes the best thing we can do is let him go homeless.

I'm struggling inside and ask her, "How do we do this in the winter with the weather dicey at best? I know he'll become a danger to the community once they turn him loose and there's no one to keep him under control, especially if he's homeless. He isn't well enough to be released, and we have no authority to detain him without the LRA. It's a horrible situation I can't believe is being forced on the community and on our family."

Our other housing option, the Elijah House, is an all-male home in the area but it isn't staffed twenty-four hours a day. Daniel can't be trusted to live in a setting where there isn't 24-hour oversight. She doesn't know if Elijah House will take Daniel given his history.

I let Karen know my concerns and hesitation about her plan. "I know he'll drink, sooner rather than later, and I don't have it in me to let him go homeless. This plan is setting me up for needing to move Daniel into our home when he does decompensate. It'll be dangerous for me, or it'll be dangerous for the community. This is a bad plan." I'm incredulous at the quick speed of his release from the hospital, and the lack of a safe plan for those of us that need to step in because the system is failing us.

I tell Karen, "How does the state hospital release him knowing he isn't well, especially when they don't have a plan in place to ensure compliance? The LRA is what gives us the ability to pull him back into the hospital for care. They need to get this in place before they let him out." I know I'm talking to a person who doesn't have it in her power to make it happen. It resides in the hands of the state mental hospital, who is doing nothing at this point. Karen feels the ideal situation would be an adult family home with 24-hour staff.

According to Karen, Daniel's new doctor will be Dr. Singh. I am so relieved that Dr. Egan will be nowhere near my son. This new doctor came to the Grace Center in July 2010. I ask her if Daniel can be in the PACT program and she says in the past he has declined. I let her know in late August Daniel said he wanted to be in the PACT program, so she agrees to check with Daniel again.

There's no way to stop the state mental hospital from releasing Daniel back into the community. The staff knows he isn't well and I know there's no way he'll comply with the rules of the Connor House because he's not stable and won't be able to follow them. When the hallucinations, delusions, and voices take over Daniel's mind, they win every time. It's not a good thing that our communities endure the dumping of state mental hospital sick people back into their home towns, why is it happening? Karen tells me they're discharging patients out of the wards due to budget constraints,[xvii] busing them back to the community they came from, and leaving them at the bus stop. A few years earlier, I sat on the board of directors for Snyder Family Treatment Center as a layperson with experience in family dynamics. I remember being alerted at one of our board meetings about the fact that patients were being bused back to our community from the State Mental Hospital, and we needed to ensure we were ready for the potential onslaught this would cause to our services? Discussions occurred regarding where we could house the homeless people after they were dropped off by the buses. The state and local mental health communities don't have the facilities or the money to take care of our mentally ill community members.[xviii] So many of the ill end up living on the streets, homeless, and become victims of violence themselves, many times they are willingly victimized.[xix,xx] When President John F. Kennedy decided to dismantle our entire mental health hospital system in the 1960s, he promised the government would fund local community facilities which would be better for the mentally ill.[xxi] Unfortunately, talk is cheap and so were the promises. The other alternative, if families aren't willing to take them back into their homes, is to dump the mentally ill out onto the streets without shelter, making it difficult to get them their medication and ensure they get enough food. Unfortunately, our situation is occurring in November and it's starting to freeze. I guess we're fortunate they're at least driving Daniel back in a van and putting him up at Connor House, even though we know he's too sick to last long under their roof.

On November 2, Daniel is discharged from the state mental hospital. He's driven by a representative of the hospital and they drop him off at the Connor House in Portland. Unfortunately, Daniel isn't consenting to using the PACT program. I'm frustrated by his reversal. He isn't concerned about getting well when he knows he's about to be free and doesn't want any hindrances on what he wants to do. The hospital discharges Daniel no better than when he arrived, even though he had nine months of inpatient hospital care both at the Grace Center and the state mental hospital. I head off to a locksmith and have two of our upstairs bedrooms fitted with locks that can only be opened from the inside. I decide to have the bedroom doors for both Karis and the master bedroom outfitted to prevent entry. A person will need to break down the door to get to the occupants. This will give law enforcement the knowledge that a forceful, violent entry occurred, if God forbid they are ever called to our home. I want to be safe, not sorry if the worst should happen. I know it's time to prepare for the chaos that will reign once again in our lives.

The Connor House is available to Daniel for up to ninety days—if he follows all the rules—even though he's still very psychotic. When Daniel arrives at the house, they lay out all of their rules and since he has been at the Connor House before, he's familiar with the layout and doesn't need a tour. Karen talks with the manager of the house and lets him know our concerns. The manager emphasizes the rules still apply and Daniel has to abide by them. I know this is an exercise in futility. I talk with the manager of the Connor House and let him know my worries. The manager tells me, "Regardless of Daniel's mental state, he must follow every rule."

"I'm worried about the open door policy and Daniel's inability to control his urges and the voices giving him direction." I'm talking to a manager who follows everything by the book and can't really do much to help with the situation. He has a system of rules to run the house and the rules are their attempt to make order out of chaos.

Unfortunately, upon arrival Daniel immediately takes to the streets and is gone all day. I stop by after work the first evening to see how he's doing and he isn't there. I know he's drinking. He has no money but that hasn't stopped him in the past.

Unfortunately, but predictably, Daniel is kicked out within three days. The Connor House calls early on the third evening and the manager tells me, "Come get Daniel because he vomited in the living room after stealing a case of beer and guzzling it all." The fact he made it three days is actually longer than I thought my paranoid schizophrenic son could manage. My heart is in flight, and I feel panic as I drive over to the Connor House. Now what do we do? It's early November, freezing cold outside, and I know Daniel can't survive on the street. He's skin and bones, and isn't dressed for the weather, this is going to end badly.

I call Karen and talk with her telling her what occurred at the home, and she advises me, "Let them kick Daniel out on the street... homeless."

"As a parent, and mother, I just can't allow this to happen." I reply. "Maybe if it was spring or summer and I didn't think he'd freeze to death or catch pneumonia I'd go that route." Karen doesn't have any other solutions to the problem.

I call my husband and let him know, "I have to go pick up Daniel." We decide to bring him home and hope for the best. My fear is at such a heightened level, and I pray, God please keep my son from hurting me.

Karen is trying to find a locked facility where Daniel can go for care since it's apparent he's intent on drinking. Karen does a great job finding a detox bed for Daniel, and two days after he's kicked out of the Connor House, crisis response detains him for drinking excessively again, and Karen takes him off to the detox facility.

I talk with Daniel and tell him, "It's sad to know you're drinking again."

"I'm sad too." He says. The look in his eyes is dejected and lost. I can tell from the tone in his voice he's very depressed. This turn of events doesn't surprise me and it's exactly what I feared would happen.

The next day, I speak with Daniel at the detox facility to check on how he's doing. He says, "My alcohol level was 0.2 before they brought me here to detox." At a level of 0.2, most people experience a blackout, having no memory of all or part of what happens during the period their blood alcohol is at this level.[xxii]

He asks, "Can I live with you guys? I don't think I can survive living on my own. I need you to help me become stable." His eyes are dark and sunken, little hope resides there.

"Dad and I will have to discuss you moving home with us, and if we decide to let you try again, you'll need to sign a contract with rules for you to abide by while under our roof."

He says, "I'm willing to do that, I'll sign your contract."

Earlier in the week, I asked Karen if I can work as Daniel's caregiver. She gets back to me and tells me, "You don't qualify for the role." What the heck, I am his mother and have been his caregiver through all of this craziness and they always discharge him into my care…how can I not be qualified? After you're hit with so many disjointed, illogical thought processes throughout the years, it seems like you finally just learn to roll over and take the hits without flinching. I'm willing to quit work and fulfill this role, if they'd allow me to, even though it would mean a very drastic wage decrease. So, now with me deemed not qualified, we're considering the possibility of hiring a care provider who'll stay with Daniel while Leonard and I are at work. The provider can help to ensure he eats, help us try to control Daniel's fluid intake, and somehow try to ensure he doesn't go off to steal beer.

During this detox stay while Daniel and I are talking, he says, "This last year when I got really bad, it was because I was under medicated, really psychotic, and drinking all the time. I know I have to take my medication and I will." I've heard all of these words before and they don't mean anything anymore.

Four days after Daniel goes inpatient at the detox facility, Karen phones me to discuss options for Daniel. She has an appointment for Daniel to meet with Shannon, his new medications nurse. She has a refill for seven days of his current medications. The Grace Center will approach him again to accept the PACT program.

"The program is willing to take him, but not at this time as they are full." Karen tells me. Some people may be graduating out of the program soon and slots may open up, but all of this is immaterial if Daniel won't agree to accept the PACT program. In the meantime, Karen and another case manager will check in on Daniel frequently.

Detox agrees to keep Daniel up to two weeks. They switch him from a detox bed to a crisis bed. I let Karen know I'm not comfortable having Daniel in our home, but I can't allow him to be homeless during the winter. I ask Karen about the possibility of a Community Options Program Entry System (COPES) provider that can be with Daniel while Leonard and I are at work. They could ensure Daniel eats, observe him, and be with him during the day. Karen says she will check into the program and get back to me. Another option Karen mentions is a group home for the mentally ill. She doesn't know if there are any openings, or what it's like at the home.

In mid-November, Karen phones to let me know, "They are discharging Daniel from detox today. There's a new state budget cut and there's no bed left for Daniel at the detox facility so he won't be able to stay for two weeks. The good news is Daniel agreed to accept the PACT program, but the bad news is there's still no opening available." First, I'm assuming the detox facility is having the same budget crunch as the state mental hospital. Secondly, the PACT program is woefully underfunded and has no room for anyone new. It's such a shame.

Karen, John, and Jamie (three different case managers) will take turns checking in with Daniel at our home on a daily basis until they can initiate the PACT program. In this way they can ensure medication compliance. Karen also lets me know it's been determined a COPES provider to help care for Daniel isn't approved. My husband will pick-up Daniel tonight from the detox facility and bring him to our home.

As soon as he arrives at our home, Leonard and I sit with Daniel and have him sign a contract with us laying out the rules which allow him to live in our home: no alcohol, medication compliance, and we'll take his car away for two years at his request. I suggest one year without a car, but he knows better and asks me to change it to two years. I'm surprised at his openness and willingness to abide by these rules, but I quickly check myself so I don't get my hopes up.

I'm sure he'll quickly break the 'no alcohol' rule. I at least feel if Daniel keeps up the alcohol and violent talk, he'll know his dad and I tried everything to allow him to stay with us if we need to kick him out. His future lies in his own hands, the hands of a paranoid schizophrenic. It seems such a sad ending to what was once the promising future he envisioned for himself when he was younger. Mental illness robs a person of all reason, logical processing, and caring about others; it's a vortex of misery and pain for all who are touched by it.

While I'm talking with Daniel the first evening, my NAMI training kicks in and I tell him, "You scare me. What we've been through with you is traumatizing to me and I don't like being alone with you." It feels good to tell him what I'm thinking and not keep it bottled up. It is healthy for me to speak the words.

Feeling more confident, I go on, "When you threaten to kill me, and do horrible things to my body, I don't even know how to respond. My whole body shuts down and I feel paralyzed. Having you around me isn't healthy for me."

I'm watching his face for any sign of violence, or anger, but he just says, "I'd never hurt you." He doesn't seem upset at my statement, and is rather nonchalant. His response is falling into line with what NAMI said to expect. What a relief.

I remind him, "You were supposed to stay 90 days at the Connor House to prove you were stable enough before you could come into our home. You only made it three days before getting kicked out." I'm internally thinking to myself, "What am I to learn from the lack of ability on his part?" Everything he's saying is just words. They have no substance.

The next evening Daniel can't sleep at all through the night. We decide that 7 AM and 7 PM will be good times to take his medicine each day. Daniel's rapidly circling the island in the kitchen muttering, talking to himself, and periodically laughing. Karis leaves the home around noon as she isn't comfortable with his behavior. I come home from work and check in on Daniel at 1 PM and bring him a sandwich from Subway. He says, "I'll try to sleep tonight."

"Please stop the caffeine so your body can come down from the stimulant." I explain to him, "A lack of sleep can cause hallucinations and delusions and you need to try and care for yourself by cutting back on caffeine so you can sleep."

There's no rhyme or reason to his need for extensive fluids. I have no idea why he craves caffeine, or even water for that matter. All I can think is it has to go back to the psychogenic polydipsia that affects some people with severe mental illness. Everything he touches seems to be to the extreme. Extreme drinking of alcohol, water, caffeine intake…nothing is ever in moderation.

The next evening after work, Daniel and I discuss a good plan for cutting back on the caffeine in his diet. We agree that in the morning before work, I'll leave a six pack of pop on the kitchen island, a baggie of ground coffee, and a brewed jug of iced tea. The rest of the caffeine I keep in the trunk of my car and bring it to work with me. While the drinks I leave for Daniel contain an insane amount of caffeine, this helps keep a lid on the total load in his system each day. He still seems internally preoccupied and while he's sitting outside smoking, you can see him laughing at things. He denies the preoccupation.

Eventually, just a few days after coming home, Daniel starts drinking and vomits all over his bed and the wall. He becomes very ill from the beer and his body immediately rejects the alcohol.

He says, "I found a five-dollar bill and walked all the way to the gas station, made the purchase, and walked back with the beer in the freezing snow."

Karis sees him hide the beer across the street in the weeds, but is at a loss of how to deal with him in such a sick state. Is she safe to confront him about the hidden beer? He remains sick all through the day. Every night before bed I take my purse upstairs and Karis does the same so I don't know where he found the money. I actually believe he walked to the store and stole the beer, but it's just a guess.

In late November, Daniel starts on a new medication for depression called Remeron and his psychiatrist and medications nurse also add a sleep aid to his regime. He sleeps all Thanksgiving Day and can't make dinner. Four days later, he says he feels better on Remeron. He's sleeping a lot and I don't know if this is normal. We ask him to join us on different excursions, but he always says no and sleeps. I worry at the level of sleeping and resting but at least when he does this I know his body is healing and repairing – and he is not stealing beer.

On December 10, 2010, I sit in on a teleconference given by two doctors: Daniel Weinberger, MD (a practicing neuroscientist and the director of Gene Cognition Research at National Institute of Mental Health for the last thirty years in Bethesda, Maryland), and Kenneth Duckworth, MD (medical director of NAMI). This teleconference is instrumental in sending me down the gene pathway for wellness. It helps solidify the information I read in 2005 from Dr. Amy Yasko. These two doctors state that while genes cause illness of the mind, there's not one gene in particular that causes schizophrenia. They believe the cancer of mental illness is schizophrenia and our genes lay out the genetic blue print of our susceptibility to inherit illness. The more accumulated genetic risk factors a person has, the higher their likelihood for schizophrenia.

The doctors claim inheritance determines the likelihood of mental illness and accumulated environmental risks increase the chance of future possibilities. They explain that our cells need to work together and our genes are the blueprint for every cells behavior. The doctors stress all gene models need to be explored in the future and doctors need to work on discovering the cellular hiccups and bottlenecks that account for risk biology. They believe in the future, there's potential for molecular targets being affected by drugs, and maybe even reversed. Doctors have learned more in the last ten years than all the years before. Researchers find syndromes with common presentations and new drugs are emerging for trials. The current drugs are just not good enough, especially for schizophrenia; they reduce symptoms but at times cause side effects which lead to the drugs needing to be stopped. The doctors ask two questions: Are the drugs neurologically effective? Do they help a patient change adaptively?

They believe the wiring in our brain isn't fixed and the local wiring can undergo some changes. These changes are a part of the study of epigenetics, which is the term used when discussing methyl groups (CH₃). Methylation acts as a switch turning the cells on and off and we can affect cellular function as needed through this mechanism.[xxiii] They go on to discuss there are four letters in the DNA genome (A, T, C, and G). The sequences differ between people, but 99% of the letters are the same, only one percent differ. They state that we receive fifty percent of our genes from each parent. Every gene is not turned on in every cell; kidney cells are not turned on in liver cells, and vice versa. Interestingly, ninety percent of schizophrenia patients start before age twenty-five, and ten percent after that. In addition, females have a later age onset than do males.[xxiv]

The doctors discuss how brain development takes time and marijuana drug use early in adolescence is linked to an increased likelihood of schizophrenia by age twenty-five. There is an illegal drug association linkage at a population level from 1 out of 100 increasing to 2 out of 100. Most people are not in danger because they only have a slightly increased genetic risk. However, people experiencing early difficulties may be alleviating symptoms by self-medicating, and marijuana facilitates the biology of the emergence of schizophrenia. They state there's clearly a statistical link. To support this, a dopaminergic and marijuana gene risk study out of New Zealand conducted by Julius Axelrod, a Nobel Prize winner, shows increased sensitivity of Catechol-O-methyl transferase (COMT) protein/enzyme effect on dopamine metabolism.[xxv] COMT is involved in neurotransmission and there's an increased schizophrenia risk of ten-fold if a person has COMT mutations and uses marijuana early in adolescence.[xxvi,xxvii]

The discussion continues with the doctors stating it takes ten years to develop a drug and get it approved by the U.S. Food and Drug Administration, and because of the length of time, pharmaceutical companies are pulling out. As they are wrapping up their talk, they let us know there is also research from the scholarly community finding a connection between Glutamate, GABA, and SAMe. I will find in the future these three items are quite impactful in the methylation pathway. The connection isn't made in their teleconference, but SAMe is the master methyl donor on the methylation pathway, which is tied to COMT. The doctors also see a pattern showing bilirubin at birth confers a small risk affect for schizophrenia.[xxviii] And finally, they haven't seen brain imaging as useful for a diagnosis of schizophrenia.

After listening to the hour and half teleconference, I'm excited to see a potential connection to my research and a tie in with Daniel. It confirms the information from Dr. Yasko, and even strengthens her research. This is a new line of thinking and very exciting for me to hear. I remember the need for Daniel to spend some time under the bilirubin lights at the hospital when he was a newborn. I remember taking him back in the first week for a stay to help clear the bilirubin buildup in his system. I also know Daniel used marijuana as an adolescent and I was instructed by his psychiatrist to let him use it and to not interfere, as he was only self-medicating. I wonder if this played a role in the beginning of his mental illness.

The information from the teleconference encourages me to continue following my own research on genetics, epigenetics, nutrigenomics and methylation. Something changed in an instant for Daniel one day in April when he was fourteen years old and I know there has to be a biochemical reason for the sudden mental shift in my son. I'm ready to rise to the challenge because I believe there may be a reason why we are going through this together as a family. There has to be a point to our suffering. This can be used to further Daniel's healing, and maybe help others someday. This goal gives me strength to put one foot in front of the other each day and inspires me to move forward. There has to be some way to rescue my son from this horrible mental illness; I'm not content to sit back and let his story unfold as it is, and I can't just kick him out of our home if he needs us. I am not going to give up on our son. I know Daniel's life holds meaning even under the most horrible conditions.

When I arrive home from work one evening, I find Daniel coughing up a lot of dark brown coffee ground looking stuff in front of the bathroom door, on the carpeting. He tried to clean it up, but since there was so much it just spread all over the carpeting. Karis came home to the situation and cleaned up the mess as best she could.

I ask Daniel, "Can you try in the future to capture the throw up in a plastic bag and put it in the refrigerator outside?" I am wondering if he has bleeding going on in his GI tract, and if I can get a sample, we can get it analyzed.

"The volume is a lot and I've been doing this for almost a year." He thinks it's tar. He continues, "I didn't tell anyone at the hospital about coughing it up." He's smirking as if this is really funny. He says the amount is increasing over time. Daniel continues to cough up the coffee ground like substance through-out the day.

I'm hoping Karen can get Daniel in to a doctor for a check-up. They'll probably want to see the stuff. I leave a text message for Karen to see if we can get him in. He doesn't have a doctor so I need Karen's help. I talk with Daniel about reducing his cigarettes to one-pack a day, and he's good with this idea.

The next morning while my husband and I are at work, Karis takes Daniel for a blood draw. However, later the same evening his health takes a turn for the worse and I end up taking Daniel to the

Providence Medical Center emergency room for acute bronchitis, cough, and gastro esophageal reflux disease.

Daniel's eyes look out of focus and glossy and I can tell he's really not well psychologically. There's a non-responsive look to his face like he's in another physical reality. This is a look I'm terribly familiar with and I know it'll lead to no good.

While we are in the ER exam room, Daniel tells me in front of the attending nurse, "You know I want to kill you."

I tell Daniel, "I know you do, you've told me before."

The nurse and I exchange looks and she's stunned to hear him just blurt it out, unprovoked as if it's always front and center in his thoughts. I try not to let my fear rise because I know it wreaks havoc on my health.

A short time later out of nowhere, he says, "I want to bludgeon blondes with a baseball bat."

The nurse looks over at me in shock and quickly leaves the room to let the staff know of the threats he's making to me. Security ends up stationed outside of his emergency room where they're monitoring his physical condition.

The nurse comes back a short time later and lets me know there's no psychiatric bed available for Daniel. "You'll need to take him home with you," she informs me. "We also checked many of our hospital options and they have no beds."

I'm stunned, but not surprised. You'd think after the medical staff heard a direct threat to me, and potentially the community, they'd be able to find a bed. There isn't much you can do when funding isn't given to this critical area. We act shocked and wonder what's going on in our communities when our mentally ill loved ones are being killed by police or hurting their own family members.

Well, we have no safe place for them, so they're on the streets or in homes where family members may not be safe.

Karen stops by the emergency room to check on us and after listening to the threats she says, "I think Daniel may be a candidate for Clozaril."

I remember back in our NAMI class when we reviewed drug options for mental illness, this was one of the drugs listed for potential use. This medication was not previously offered to us. I remember our teacher in the class saying her son was on this medication and she thinks it's a great drug and was really successful in treating her son's schizophrenia.

"Do you mind if I leave to head over to Grace Center and see about getting Daniel accepted into the Clozaril program?" Karen asks.

I nod. "Yes, please do anything you can to help." I see Daniel's future dimming by the day. We can't find lasting help and we're quickly coming to an end where I see no promise and no hope. Karen leaves me in the emergency room and I bring Daniel home later that evening with no positive progress and no optimism for change. I pray God will keep my son from harming me and place a hedge of protection all around our home.

# Chapter Fifteen:

# Hope Renewed – January 2011

———◆———

*Healing is a matter of time, but it is sometimes also a matter of opportunity.*
*Hippocrates*

On January 3, 2011, we find out Daniel is approved for admission to the Clozaril program. This medication's been around since the 1970s but was pulled off the market due to some deaths in patients whose leukocytes (white blood cells) and neutrophils (a type of white blood cell) plummeted so they couldn't fight off infections.[xxix] It's an atypical antipsychotic used for people with treatment resistant schizophrenia who don't respond well to at least two standard antipsychotics because they have intolerable side effects, or because they were insufficiently effective.[xxx] Clozaril can significantly reduce symptoms of schizophrenia so the patient has fewer hospitalizations. It can increase the patient's enjoyment in life and improve their level of functioning. It's been proven to be superior to standard antipsychotics.[xxxi]

Karen lays out the program for Daniel and he's assigned a new nurse, Donna, to manage the new medication. She manages and monitors all patients on Clozaril at the Grace Center because the program is quite stringent. Many agency's need to sign off on the results of Daniel's blood work to ensure his blood tests show his neutrophils are in an acceptable range before they fill his prescription each week. The groups involved in authorizing the medication include the lab that draws the blood, the psychiatrist who reviews the results, the pharmacy that fills the prescription, and the National Clozaril Registry. All of the groups have to agree

Daniel's blood levels are adequate to tolerate the medication before he gets a refill.

Donna tells us Daniel needs a blood draw each week to check his white blood cell count (immune system cells that protect our bodies from invaders) and his neutrophil count (immune system cells that respond to inflammation). His blood draw results are then reviewed by the four groups. If his blood levels are accepted by all four, he'll receive a one-week supply. We need to follow this same process each week until he's been on Clozaril for six months with good blood levels. From there we can move to a blood draw every two weeks. At the end of one year of stability, and if all the blood levels have stayed in a normal range, he can switch to once a month blood draws.

I'm hopeful as Donna explains she has seen very good results for the patients whose body systems can tolerate the medication. "Some patients find great relief in the cessation of the desire to drink alcohol," she tells us.

I'm hopeful this medication will be a game changer. Daniel immediately gets a blood draw and we wait to make sure he's a candidate with his health history and the blood level results. Everything comes back okay and we're given the green light to start him on Clozaril.

It seems like a miracle because three days later Daniel is sober and he has little or no drive for alcohol. I'm tempted to pinch myself as this seems too good to be true. In my quiet time I ask God to keep my son responding to this drug in a healthy way and keep his blood levels stable.

When you're in such a deep, despairing hole where nothing looks like it can get better, you have to choose to hold on to faith, or walk away and declare it a sham. Both are hard to endure. I realize even though I have such anger at God for no healing reprieve, I have to learn to stand up and take responsibility for my part in my son's health. Every step on this walk has been fraught with such turmoil and fear and it would've been easier to put up the walls, push out my faith… But of all the steps we took, the hardest was holding on to God and letting him guide me in compassion and wisdom.

Daniel's surprised at the quick turn-around in his craving for alcohol. We're all in shock at this profound, immediate change. My happiness turns to questions: Why are we just now trying this drug? Why wasn't Daniel placed on this program earlier? Why not at the state mental hospital when he was there for so long? Could we have stabilized him years before and saved him from so many brain damaging episodes of psychosis and seven hospitalizations? Don't get me wrong, we're thrilled at the results and that Daniel is finally on this medication, but we are left wondering, 'why the wait?'

Even though the alcohol cravings are subsiding, Daniel still deals with delusions, hallucinations, voices, pacing the driveway outside, laughing and responding to the voices, and circling the kitchen island incessantly. I know this will take time and the healing process is going to be slow. It's such a relief to not worry about coming home from work and finding Daniel drinking. It's nice to know he won't be out stealing alcohol to get his fix.

A few months into the Clozaril program, Daniel's blood tests for his white blood cell counts and neutrophils levels aren't looking very good. We spend months adjusting the dose and worrying each week about how his blood will check out. We hit a point where we start lowering the Clozaril dose because his white blood cell and neutrophil levels are falling dangerously low and we may need to wean him off of the medication. Thinking of them dropping Daniel off of Clozaril fills me with immense fear. Daniel is two months sober and this is truly a miracle, we just need his body to adjust to this medication and stabilize and allow time for the hallucinations, delusions, and voices to end.

Daniel's body takes more than ten months to stabilize his white blood cell count before we can move to a blood draw every two weeks. Every time his blood work drops into a bad range, we're back at square one trying to get a continuous stable six-month period. Slowly he begins to stabilize.

During these ten months I take Daniel each week for blood draws and we continue to give Clozaril time to adjust in his system. He still has no cravings for alcohol and we're starting to breathe more easily, less on edge waiting for a crisis. Karen sets us up with a general practitioner for Daniel, someone to help us with the struggles in Daniel's physical body. Unfortunately, we learn we'll soon lose Karen as Daniel's case manager. She receives a much deserved promotion to another job within the psychiatric system. This is a tough loss as Karen is such a great support resource for me during rough times and she'll be sorely missed as our advocate in the mental health system. She knows our struggles and our hopes and has become a big part of bringing health to our son. She'll leave a huge void for someone else to fill.

Daniel and I like his new general practitioner, Dr. West. He's very thorough in assessing Daniel's health and it's obvious he's listening to Daniel's history and isn't taken aback by the psychiatric situation. When I bring up methylation and the possibility of Daniel's mutations, he pulls open his laptop and begins researching the topic and is open to helping me with future testing for Daniel. This doctor will be a very welcome addition to our medical team. Sometimes you can tell when you've found an open minded physician who will help you dig deep for answers, and I think we've found just the right one for Daniel.

Daniel has now successfully been on Clozaril for ten months and after talking with him about genetic mutations and the methylation cycle, Daniel is open to the option of testing for his methylation cycle mutations. I've been waiting for Daniel to be willing to get these tests since he was in the state mental hospital. Since I learned Tyler, Karis, and I had MTHFR mutations, I was sure Daniel did to. In my studies, I learned the methylation pathway is a key biochemical pathway in our body and is tied to cellular function. Every cell in our body needs to be able to methylate. If mutations occur in this critical pathway your body cannot function as well, which puts you at risk for health issues.[xxxii] There are key neurotransmitters that depend on an adequately functioning methylation cycle.[xxxiii]

I wonder what Daniel's genes look like, are they mutated? In the past he was never open to any suggestions of testing of any kind to see if we could find an underlying disorder behind his struggles. This is another positive step made possible by the Clozaril medication. One of the mutations on the methylation pathway is MTHFR and Dr. West runs the blood test on Daniel. The results show Daniel has two heterozygous mutations for A1298T and C677T (they call this compound heterozygous). This genotype is associated with hyperhomocysteinemia and an increased risk for coronary artery disease and venous thrombosis (blood clots).[xxxiv]

Dr. West starts Daniel on Fola Pro (Vitamin B9-Folate…not folic acid) and he builds up to ten tablets a day, then switches over to Deplin (a prescription dose of 7.5 mg L-5 methyltetrahydrofolate). A month after we make the switch to Deplin, Daniel spirals into a psychosis, and we lose a lot of positive ground we made during the last ten months. He becomes very angry, and the positive symptoms of schizophrenia are increased. Positive symptoms aren't actually positive. Daniel's psychiatrist explains positive symptoms as traits added to his personality that aren't normal in healthy individuals.[xxxv] We talk with Dr. West at the next appointment and decide Daniel needs to stop Deplin because he must have mutations either upstream or downstream on his methylation cycle and I need to figure out which ones are causing him issues.

When I get home, I immediately get online and order a genetic test kit from Dr. Amy Yasko at Holisticheal.com. She tests for thirty single nucleotide polymorphisms (SNPs) which she considers important to address, and which reside in key areas of the methylation pathway. In addressing these SNPs, we help the methylation cycle function well in our cells by giving them the specific nutrients they need. I know I can't experiment on Daniel because he's so fragile, and so I'll try this process on me first to learn if there are down sides to this new approach.

I too have neurological issues and received a multiple sclerosis diagnosis when I was thirty years old. My story is its own odyssey, but I know I also need to tackle my health issues and I'm sure I'll find they're tied to the methylation pathway as well. When I was diagnosed with multiple sclerosis, I had five lesions in my brain, spread over both brain hemispheres. I decide to use myself as a guinea pig to see if healing the methylation pathway brings me any relief before I turn my attention to working on Daniel. He's so fragile and I don't want to cause him to slip further into psychosis by trying this on him first. If I work on myself, I am able to discern the slightest positive or negative reaction as I work through the process. I'm hoping if I am successful on myself, I can then start the process with Daniel.

I'm excited the day the DNA test kit arrives from Dr. Yasko. I poke my finger and collect three small blood drops on a felt cloth and let it air dry, then ship it back to the lab. Now I wait and hope the results shed some light on my mutated genes and see what my husband and I may have passed on to Daniel. I know he has major methylation issues from how sick he became so quickly when he started Deplin.

When I bought the genetic test from Dr. Yasko, I also received free books and study guides to read and learn about methylation while I wait the three months for the results. She also has free videos on her website that teach on the methylation pathway. There's a lot to understand about the methylation cycle and I'm eager to see if I can find a pattern to this madness. I spend the next three months reading and trying to absorb what Dr. Yasko is teaching. She's so brilliant that I need to read and reread sections over and over again to understand them.

While we're waiting for my methylation results, Daniel tells Dr. West he's having a hard time swallowing; his heart is beating quite rapidly and his weight is falling. "It feels like something is stuck in my throat so I can only eat certain foods."

He now eats only really soft foods so they won't get stuck. Daniel is now a vegan and will only eat certain food items so he's hardly consuming any calories, protein or fats. Daniel's weight is down to 135 pounds and since he's five feet eleven inches tall, the doctor is concerned about how thin he's becoming.

Dr. West sends us to a gastroenterologist, Dr. Bell, who orders a bedside swallow test to be performed at a local hospital. After completing the test, Dr. Bell says, "The swallowing difficulty may be

caused by Clozaril and Daniel may need to stop the medication."
The thought of this new doctor pushing to take Daniel off Clozaril
makes me freeze up inside. He has no idea the hell we've endured.
My mind is in turmoil and I can't think.

Daniel immediately says, "Absolutely not, I won't stop the
medication."

My fear is Dr. Bell can push the situation and notify Daniel's
psychiatric team of the need to discontinue Clozaril and we'll have
no way to fight the determination. The drug is so heavily regulated
that if you're taken off the drug for any reason, you can never be put
back on. We can't let this happen.

Dr. Bell informs me, "I want you to start feeding Daniel via a
tube which you'll put down his nose at night." Daniel is shaking his
head no.

"If Daniel is that ill, he should be hospitalized until he's stable."
I continue. "Daniel isn't psychologically well enough to grasp the
situation and he won't allow me to intubate him for feedings at
night."

The doctor is making a note of my refusal to do the procedure
on Daniel so if he dies, he is clear of any wrong doing. The doctor
tells me, "I won't admit Daniel to the hospital for care."

I turn to Daniel and ask him, "Will you allow me to feed you via
a tube while you're sleeping?" Again, he resolutely refuses.

That evening, Karis and I are visiting on the phone and she tells
me, "You need to have Daniel write down his refusal of the doctor's
request and have him list what he'll allow them to do and have him
sign the document."

I go to Daniel again and talk with him about what the doctor wants to do each night while he's sleeping to help him gain weight. He again says, "No way."

I give him some paper and a pen. "Please write down your desires so if you die the state can't come after our family for not force feeding you." It sounds so cold and harsh, but we're living in a cold harsh reality. If I can't get my son to comply, then I have to protect our family. I file his note to the side and pray I never have to use it in a court of law.

Two months go by and Daniel's rapidly losing weight. I can't get him to eat anything containing calories and his weight is now at 120 pounds. His gastroenterologist still wants to put a feeding tube down his throat. I tell the doctor again, "If Daniel needs this kind of care, you should put him in the hospital where people can take care of the psychiatric and emotional issues that are plaguing him."

I continue, "His not eating is obviously coming off a psychiatric problem as we've ruled out a physical issue for the feeling of chocking. Daniel's afraid he's fat and has a body image issue where he fears every pound he gains," I add in frustration.

We're at a standstill and I start to feel if Daniel dies at this point it'll be a relief to him from these last two decades of misery and suffering. There are worse things in life than physical death. Dying definitely brings closure to situations and I know I've fought the good fight to get care for our son and make sure he's sheltered to the best of our ability. It would be a lie to say I'm not tired. I am so exhausted and the fight has been going on too long; however, I see a ray of light in the Clozaril medication and the end of Daniel's alcohol addiction.

I know we don't have all of the answers and I have some promising research I have been following, but I'm still waiting for my genetic mutation test results from Dr. Yasko. I finally have Daniel at a place where he'll work with me on this new area of research regarding nutrigenomics, epigenetics, and the methylation pathway. I hold great hope in this being very important in getting him better.

Even though Daniel is sober, he's still stuck in certain thinking loops which are difficult to break. The hallucinations, delusions, and voices still own his mind. I know there's more that needs to be done to orient him to reality and as Daniel continues to improve off of alcohol. I'm waiting for the time to discuss these options as a means to recovering his mind once the genetic results arrive.

We're very fortunate that Daniel finally comes out of his eating disordered thinking on his own, but it still takes a few months. We did nothing to make this happen from a medical standpoint. It appears he just chose to change his thinking. Maybe the voices were winning during the time period and bringing condemnation and humiliation to him, and for some reason they changed their focus onto a new diversion. His weight slowly rises over the next few months until he weighs in at 138 pounds. This change brings me great relief but we don't know why or what triggered his thinking to switch. He's still listening to voices and a derogatory internal monologue which makes him feel inferior.

Daniel's health is improving every month he spends on Clozaril and off of alcohol. I wonder if this is what enabled the eating disorder to remedy itself. The voices, hallucinations, and delusions are still a problem but you have to take victory in whatever struggles are overcome. This brings such an overwhelming sense of peace that I'm afraid to embrace it. What if this reprieve is fleeting, or if the drinking alcohol and not eating start back up?

Daniel turns thirty years old in 2011 which is a huge celebration and I think back on him always telling me he would be dead by age 30. I feel such relief that he made it to this age and has not given up his fight. When I look at Daniel, I am filled with such wonder and pride. He shows me what God's grace looks like. We're all relevant and needed in someone's life. I know I have a purpose and a mission to fulfill while I'm here, and I pray for strength each day to be wise and know what steps are needed to continue to bring healing to my son.

# CHAPTER SIXTEEN:

## Keep My Son Receptive

———◆———

*He that will not apply new remedies must expect new evils; for time is the greatest innovator.*
*Francis Bacon*

When my DNA methylation SNP results come in, I find I have eleven mutations out of the thirty. Three of the mutations are double mutations and two of those three are the COMT V158M and COMT H62H. These two mutations affect brain neurotransmitters and I think maybe, just maybe I am on to something. I remember many years back listening to the two neuroscientists speak on COMT and its tie to schizophrenia. If I have double mutations on these two SNP sites, then I know I for sure passed on a mutation to our son. The third double mutation is on VDR Taq which affects vitamin D receptors and dopamine levels. It's interesting that I have neurological issues and an MS diagnosis and have double mutations on neurotransmitters. Coincidence or linked?

I start applying the Yasko protocol to myself and I find my own symptoms of neurological pain, muscle spasticity, electrical shocks, and numbness easing as time goes on. My thinking is if I can follow the information and see improvement in myself, I can convince Daniel to allow me to try the protocol on him because he'll see the improvement I'm making with my own medical issues. His health is so delicate I don't want to mess up the progress we've made to date with the Clozaril medication.

Daniel sees the improvement in my health as the months go by and decides he'll allow me to do a DNA test on him. I expected a bigger battle, but we both saw my improvement so it was easy for him to say yes. I don't think this would've been possible if he had not been sober from the Clozaril medication. I am so thankful for his case manager making the recommendation back in the hospital to submit his name as a possible candidate for the drug. I'm also thankful for his awesome medications nurse for working with us in implementing the Clozaril program. His psychiatric team is truly helping him. I am now intrigued to see what we'll find in Daniel's testing, but am hesitant because of his backward progression when we tried Deplin. I decide to just go for it and order the blood test from Dr. Yasko. When the DNA test kit comes in, Daniel doesn't hesitate to poke his finger and give me three blood drops on the felt cloth. I feel such excitement when I mail off the sample. I wish there was a way to reduce the wait time.

As we wait for Daniel's test results, I still notice he's laughing and interacting with something when he thinks he's alone. I don't know if I should be worried or if I'm just imagining the situation. To confirm my fears will mean he's still seeing, hearing, and walking around in a state of confusion. Karis mentions on some of her visits that she sees him conversing with himself when he thinks no one is looking. I hate to even entertain the thought that Daniel's still hearing voices. I am just too exhausted to want to know, so I don't ask him. I feel like those three mystic monkeys, 'see no evil, hear no evil, speak no evil.' I just put up my blinders and wait. I hope Clozaril keeps on doing its job and keeps him stabile enough that the alcohol struggle stays a non-issue. Since Daniel's been on the Clozaril medication, we haven't made any emergency room runs, he hasn't been hospitalized, and there hasn't been any need for inpatient detox for alcohol intoxication.

In early 2012, Daniel's improving in great part because his drunken binges are over. This change in the situation allows me to get back to genetic mutations research and to continue learning this new field of methylation cycle function. As I research, I'm learning about epigenetics and methylation and how every cell has to be able to donate and accept methyl groups ($CH_3$ molecule) to aid enzymes and substrates.[xxxvi] The function of methylation is to turn on and off genes (which is another term for epigenetics) which enables cells to process chemicals and toxins (biotransformation) into less harmful water-soluble substances so they can be excreted, build neurotransmitters (dopamine, serotonin, epinephrine, and norepinephrine), process hormones, build immune cells (NT cells, Natural Killer cells), enable DNA and RNA synthesis, produce energy (CoQ10, carnitine, ATP), and build protective coating on nerves (myelination).

I learn that our genes are organized into chromosomes and there are 23 chromosome pairs that we inherit from our mother and father for a total of 46 genome chromosomes. When various letter combinations (A, T, C, or G) are left out, re-ordered, or substituted, this creates a Single Nucleotide Polymorphism (SNP). There are ten million SNPs that have the potential to affect our health.[xxxvii,xxxviii] I find a person can change the deck they've been dealt at birth and bypass mutations to get the methylation cycle working adequately. This is done by giving the system special cofactors and other nutrients it is lacking at certain points in the cycle. Methylation is genetically inherited and trans-generational; you can pay now or pay later if you chose to not address mutations on the methylation pathway.[xxxix] If the methylation cycle can be made to perform successfully, chronic conditions can be improved and the process to recover the pathway can begin. What works nutrient wise for one person may not work for another because we each have our own unique genetic blueprint, environmental exposures, heavy metal toxicity, gut function, stress, diet, and viral, bacterial, microbial, and parasitic loads.[xl]

When we receive Daniel's methylation pathway SNP mutation results, we find he has ten mutations out of the thirty tested. He has double mutations on both COMT SNPs just like I do, along with the double mutation on VDR Taq too.

Now I can see a reason why Daniel has neurotransmitter issues which lead to mental health problems. When combined with his environmental toxic load (poor diet, poor sleep, poor digestion, toxins from smoking, alcohol stripping out nutrients, and marijuana risk associated with COMT genes) and his predisposition to issues because of his SNPs, it's easy see where the problems intersect. Our next step is to take his SNP results and map them out on the methylation pathway diagram given to us from Dr. Yasko. After doing this we're able to determine the order for adding supplements and chose our nutrient options that Dr. Yasko lists in her chart. This is a far different approach than what we attempted when we just turned on the MTHFR wheel by adding Deplin (L-5 Methyltetrahydrofolate).

I take Daniel to his next psychiatric appointment and give the medications nurse (Donna) a copy of all of the results of his genetic testing. I walk Donna through the protocol and let her know my plans for slowly adding the nutrients specific to his mutations. We won't be changing his pharmaceutical prescriptions because they are felt to be necessary for his stability. The way I see it, the psychiatric medications aren't stopping the hallucinations, delusions, or voices so I'll just ignore them and move on with working on his methylation pathway. I let Donna know, "Each time Daniel comes to an appointment, he'll give you an updated list of nutrients he's on so you can know what nutrients he's taking." The nutrients may be cofactors, amino acids, enzymes, vitamins, probiotics, or minerals, etc. The supplements are specific to Daniel's needs based on his methylation mutations. Donna will make note of what Daniel is on, and how his behavior is improving or degrading at each visit.

The psychiatric team is on board with the process but they tell me, "Don't get your hopes up for success as many people have held out hope for other ideas in the past and they didn't come to fruition, which is a devastating let down."

"This seems really right to me," I tell Donna. "We're tackling the healing of Daniel's body at the cellular level. The theory is that when the cellular function heals over time, his body will respond and his symptoms will slowly recede. As the cells are working more efficiently the body will begin the healing process." I feel really good about this approach and it makes sense.

That evening I also ask Daniel, "Watch how you feel each time you add another supplement to your daily regime. You need to watch for anger, anxiety, sleep issues, addiction cravings, depressions, and psychosis, and I'll be watching you too." I'm watching for any changes in behavior which will alert me to the fact we need to slow down adding supplements, reduce the dose, or remove the nutrient. I have his old behavior issues ingrained in my memory.

Now that we have Daniel's results, I need to get smart on the process for interpreting the results and how to implement the Yasko protocol before we start the process on Daniel. To do this, I ask Leonard to take me to Maine to sit through a conference with Dr. Yasko so she can teach us about the program and be available for questions and answers. I decide to hold off on implementing anything other than some of the Step One foundational supplements for Daniel until I can learn more from Dr. Yasko. I sit through a three-day conference with Dr. Yasko so I can learn and ask questions. I am so excited for this journey because I know deep inside this is the answer. It makes too much sense to ignore the potential gains made by going down this pathway. The trip is also a great time to be alone with Leonard and talk about our hopes and dreams. Will Daniel be able to get a job, have his own home, and a family? Will we ever live in a time where we don't fear suicide and the dreaded knock on the door in the middle of the night? We walk along the pier and eat great seafood and pray this new research turns our lives around.

It turns out to be a really wise choice to go to the conference. I find the stories of other parents struggling to recover their children from autism, chronic fatigue syndrome, neurological issues, and poor mitochondrial function fascinating. It's amazing to think the methylation pathway is so far reaching in the symptoms and illnesses that come off of SNP mutations on the various wheels and locations. The more mutations in this critical pathway, the harder it is for the body to function optimally.

We check in with Daniel daily to make sure he's okay. This is a real test because we left him home alone. In the past when we left Daniel, he always fell apart and frantic calls would come my way. We ask Tyler if he'll please check in on Daniel and visit often so he doesn't feel alone. Daniel knows we're doing this trip for him so we can learn how to get him well. He's embracing this process and is eager for us to learn. This change in his thinking is so different from the years past when I couldn't get him to listen because he felt he was fine. Now with the help of Clozaril giving him sobriety, he's able to embrace this journey and is hoping for the best right along with us.

The conference is very informative and I'm able to personally ask some questions of Dr. Yasko regarding my own health struggles. Having dealt with neurological issues since I was thirty years old, the allopathic doctors just made me more and more sick over the course of five years of treatment. I ended up walking away from allopathic care and their massive steroids and sought out a functional medical doctor (Richard Wilkinson, MD) who worked with me on a nutritional, holistic approach instead of man-made synthetic medications. This decision was crucial to my healthier functioning today. I no longer walk with a cane. I said no to a wheel chair and I never looked back.

It's interesting when Dr. Yasko asks me, "Do you live near a nuclear reservation? Because of the heavy metal toxicity (uranium, cadmium and lead) in your system, your profile mirrors what I've seen in others living near nuclear sites." She has no way of knowing that I indeed live downstream of a nuclear reservation. I feel this methylation protocol will heal both me and Daniel of our long term health issues. I also know that anything I learn here I can share with other family members that may very well carry the same genetic methylation issues Daniel and I do. I know with my family history of mental illness, this train of reasoning is crucial to all the generations both past, present and future.

# CHAPTER SEVENTEEN:

# Keep My Son Improving

———◆———

*Faith is a knowledge within the heart, beyond the reach of proof.*
*Khalil Gibran*

We return from Dr. Yasko's conference and I can't wait to start implementing the process. In October 2012, I finally start Dr. Yasko's protocol for Daniel. I start with baby steps, implementing the supplements specific to each mutation in a specific order. Dr. Yasko let us know this isn't so much a sprint as it is a marathon. Things will take time and we need to be patient.

Upon returning from the conference, I begin implementing the supplementation for Daniel, dependent directly on his methylation mutation SNPs. The results from Dr. Yasko include a supplementation listing of possible choices of different supplements that address the specific mutations. The listing gives multiple supplement options for each SNP of which you can choose the one you want to start with. You don't choose all of them. I find many of the supplements give support to multiple SNPs. When I add B12 for one mutation, it also causes an increase in functional ability in another location on the methylation pathway. So I have to be careful and watch Daniel for symptoms of aggression, anger, depression, anxiety, insomnia, and isolation. Dr. Yasko's protocol is very nutrient intensive, listing numerous supplements which aid the enzyme formation at the SNP site. I don't follow her protocol exactly as I was selective on the amounts of nutrients added, and didn't add them all as many people state you should do.

We begin the long, slow process of layering in nutrients and watching Daniel for adverse reactions. The months pass and Daniel's showing gradual improvement. Clozaril is still keeping his alcohol addiction in check and he's still alcohol free since January 2011. He's feeling less anxious and angry with each addition made in his nutrients. It is slow going, but Daniel and I are seeing changes that are really positive. The months keep ticking by and we have no backward negative movement in Daniels behavior. Each month is better than the month before. We keep Donna updated each month.

In January 2013, we give Daniel his car back after the two-year contract period ends because he's still sober. I keep talking about miracles, but Daniel is two years sober, an impressive feat for him. From drinking such huge volumes of alcohol and battling paranoid schizophrenia to sobriety and approaching sanity, our family is absolutely elated. Tyler is starting to let his guard down around Daniel and is warming up to the idea that Daniel is beginning to improve and is getting better.

In August 2013, Daniel reinstates his standing at the community college so he can take classes again. He signs up for a class, but prior to the start of the quarter he decides to drop the class and concentrate on his health and returning his body chemistry to normal. I'm impressed he realizes on his own that the potential stress could throw off his progress. I think when the voices are silenced, and have been quiet for some time, he'll be ready to tackle college again. I encourage him to not feel bad about himself for not having a bachelor's degree. He should be so proud of himself for completing his Associate of Arts degree while suffering from mental illness. We know how smart he is; he has nothing to prove to anyone.

In the autumn of 2013, Daniel goes to the rescue of his dad, Ellen, and Rose (Tyler's two daughters) when they find themselves stranded with car problems. It's so nice to have him in such an improved state of health such that he's now coming to the aid of family members. I am out of town and Leonard doesn't hesitate to contact Daniel to come and pick them up, help them get the car towed, and bring everyone home safely. He's taking a bigger and bigger role in the family. I give him my grocery list and debit card and he makes all of the purchases. I'm finding I am no longer going to the grocery store and Daniel is capable of filling that function for me. In the past I never would have given him my debit card for fear he would purchase alcohol…in fact, I never gave him any form of currency to purchase anything. The times they are a changing!

One year in on the protocol (October 2013) and amazingly Daniel starts working on his math skills again. I even find him working on geometry at the kitchen table. I talk to him periodically about trying to read to see if his ability to read and retain is improving. After a couple days' time, he sets the books aside and I tell him that it's okay. He lost the ability to read and retain over a decade ago but I'm confident the healing will happen.

"Don't push yourself, just relax and flow with the healing," I tell him. The simple fact he picked up the math and reading material is amazing. They are small signs of progress and I see them as crucial stepping stones to recovery.

Daniel lets me know that after the first year of the protocol he no longer has hallucinations, and the delusional thinking is starting to subside. As the months keep ticking by, it's becoming apparent something huge is changing in his mind and in his health. Everyone around him sees the transformation.

Tyler notices the changes in Daniel too and recognizes he's starting to see his brother coming back to us again. I really didn't think we'd ever see the day where he would let down his guard and allow his daughters back around Daniel. I no longer get calls from Tyler asking me where I am and if I'm at the house because Leonard has the girls and he doesn't want the girls at the house if I'm not also there. Those days are gone.

One evening, Daniel calls me at work. "I'm just checking on you to make sure you're okay. You're late coming home and I was worried." I'm stunned to hear him say this because he's caring about someone other than himself for the first time since he was fourteen years old.

"I'm just working a bit longer, but I'm heading home shortly," I let him know. After we hang up, I shut my office door and cry. I cry in happiness that he cares about others again, for the healing our family is seeing, and for the alleviation of the tremendous fear I lived under for so long. What may seem so normal for other families is a huge milestone for ours. Two decades later, we're seeing signs of our son again. I pick up the phone and call my husband to let him know of the change in Daniel. The words come out between happy tears as I tell Leonard about the phone call. We're both in shock, but in a good way for once. I never thought my son would phone me and check up on me to make sure I'm well.

I know this methylation pathway process is healing Daniel's body. All of the changes happening are so exciting and they're compounding one on top of the other. I hope Daniel has a future and I wonder if this can really be happening, but I keep my hopes in check and wait because I don't know if it will continue, or what hardships may await us.

We see Daniel start to show an interest in hygiene. It's becoming more important to him and he sets up a schedule for himself to make sure he brushes, bathes, and cares for himself on a regular basis. He's also doing household chores, cooking his own meals, and buying his own groceries, which is huge for him. He leaves the house and drives to buy groceries and then comes home and cooks his own meals. He's still a vegan and is quite particular about what he eats. He stands at the grocery aisle shelf and reads the labels for content. Leonard and I smile when we notice how important the content of each can are and we're joyful to see him have such an interest in what he's putting into his body because he's now invested in his health. He's embracing feeling well and rejoining life again. It's like he was mentally stunted at age 14 when he first became sick and is beginning to mature, as if he's just now growing into an adult.

# CHAPTER EIGHTEEN:

# Keep My Son Free from Voices

————◆————

*Faith consists in believing when it is beyond the power of reason to believe.*
*Voltaire*

It's November 2013, one year after implementing the methylation protocol, and I'm shocked to find out Daniel still hears voices but can filter them and he knows they aren't real. Tyler is discussing issues with Daniel one afternoon at the house regarding me potentially writing this book. In the discussions, Tyler asks Daniel the questions I never do. Why don't I, am I afraid of the answers?

I'm devastated to hear the voices aren't gone and I find myself resenting the question was asked. It's nice to walk around presuming the best and not wanting to know the worst, then you don't have to deal with the disappointment of finding out the voices are still there. In my mind, this presents a problem. I know Daniel has improved tremendously, but I want to heal my son to a point where he has silence in his brain and isn't having to filter out voices to be present with us. I know we'll keep on implementing the nutrients that will heal Daniel's methylation cycle and eventually, given enough time, he'll have his brain to himself. To see him now compared to 2010 is a miracle. I'm elated and I feel safe. It's wonderful to see Daniel with eyes that are clear and taking in life and his surroundings.

In December 2013, my mom (whom I moved to town in August 2013) is becoming very ill and she won't allow any treatment to save her life. Daniel is so kind and compassionate towards her. He goes every evening to her assisted living apartment to take her out front to smoke. This is the one thing that brings mom happiness and he wants to be sure she's feeling calm before bed. The facility management hates that we take her out to smoke but I let them know her days are few and if this gives her peace, I see nothing wrong with the smoke breaks.

I hire extra support from the caregivers at her apartment to take her out three times a day to smoke and Daniel says he'll take her out twice in the evening, once after dinner and once before bed. It gives mom peace and she calms down. My mom loves spending time with Daniel and is glad she has the opportunity to get to know him as a healthy young man. She frequently says how happy she is to see him doing so well. Daniel keeps going every night without fail until her passing. He's come so far in his ability to reason, think of others, show compassion, and be part of the community. It makes me so proud of the huge strides he's made. He never gave up and survived much more than I think I possibly could. In early January, we lose mom and she's finally at peace. She had many strokes and heart issues just as the rest of her family did, the same health issues that are linked on the methylation pathway. I ran the SNP testing on mom too, but she didn't want to fight any more to stay alive so we didn't try to implement any positive nutrient changes.

In April 2014, Daniel goes to Dr. West for what appears to be blood in his urine. Daniel has testing done, including an ultrasound of his bladder and kidneys. All the test results are normal. There's no blood in his urine and no issues with his organs. I recall learning of Pyrrole Disorder which causes urine to turn red on exposure to UV rays. I spend some time researching and reading about Pyrrole Disorder to see if it sounds like Daniel. A large percentages of schizophrenics have this illness, as do many people with other

mental disorders.<sup>xli</sup> Daniel has some of the symptoms and so I talk
with him about his willingness to get this disorder tested the next
time he sees Dr. West.  He's open to the idea so I put into motion
the request for a lab slip from his doctor.  I learn Daniel will need
to stop zinc and vitamin B6 for two weeks prior to the testing.  If
Daniel finds out he has Pyrrole Disorder, the remedy consists of
large doses of Zinc, P5P (B6), Omega 6, Vitamin C, Vitamin E, and
Evening Primrose oil.

His test results come back normal and I'm disappointed.  I was
hoping the disorder might be affecting him and maybe we could
silence the voices by treating this illness.  I resolve myself to being
patient as we follow the protocol for his methylation issues.  It takes
time, and as Dr. Yasko always says, this is a marathon, not a sprint.
It's hard to go slow and be patient but we've made so much progress
that I know this is the answer and we're on the right track to
recovering Daniel's sanity.

Daniel and I continue to add supplements slowly over time and
in July 2014, we add magnesium to his list of nutrients.  We also
spend time looking at the supplements he's taking to address his
different mutations and decide to split them out over five different
times in the day so he isn't taking them all at the same time before
bed.  I know from my research that Vitamin A should be taken apart
from Vitamin D because they both are taken up by the same cell
receptor.  We split these apart on the new phased chart.  I also know
to take zinc apart from calcium and iron to aid in its absorption.
Integrating this information, we come up with a new plan for
phasing the nutrients in over the day to help with absorption and
utilization of the supplements.

In September 2014, my husband and Daniel fly to Florida to see
me and stay a week.  I left a week earlier to enjoy some time with

my girlfriend and old boss, Pam, and I'm excited to see the guys. Daniel travels surprisingly well even though he used to have issues with anxiety about going to new places or flying on a plane. He enjoys the new experience of swimming in the Gulf of Mexico. This is remarkable for any paranoid schizophrenic because they do not like leaving their comfort zone and going places they don't feel secure. He's changing and improving by leaps and bounds and the effect is profound. Daniel really enjoys swimming in the Gulf and riding the waves. He's hesitant at first, but when he sees how far out I can walk with the water still only up to my waist, he steps in. He takes to it like a fish. It's wonderful seeing him tanned and happy in a new environment.

When we return from Florida, we decide to add another supplement. I know with winter coming on we should add zinc to his supplements so we can get his immune system strong for the winter. Daniel is still a smoker and each winter he gets a bad cough. He's now on fourteen supplements and I think unless something changes drastically, we are at a point where we can maintain these and let some time go by to see how he continues to do mentally. We keep an eye out for adverse reactions, but everything appears to be great and there are no issues with the addition of zinc.

Daniel's new listing of supplements are:

- ◆ Adenosyl B-12 L-5 methyl tetrahydrofolate (Fola Pro)
- ◆ Hydroxy B-12 drops
- ◆ sublingual tablet
- ◆ Multi-vitamin (All-in-One)
- ◆ Vitamin B-150
- ◆ ACAT/BHMT Compounded

- Probiotics

- Wobenzyme N (Pancreatic enzymes)

- Digestive Enzymes

- GABA

- TMG

- SAMe

- Vitamin $D_3$

- Magnesium

- Zinc

# CHAPTER NINETEEN:

# Keep My Son's Mind at Peace

———◆———

*A quiet mind cureth all.*
*Robert Burton*

I am sitting one day in late September 2014 working on this book and I casually ask Daniel, "Do you still hears voices?" I hold my breath. This is a huge step for me because most of the time I'm afraid to know the answers to these types of questions, but I know something seems different with him. His demeanor, the way he was able to travel to Florida and try new things is profound and unusual.

To my surprise he answers, "I haven't heard any voices in two months."

I sit stunned and shocked. I want to burst into tears because my spirit is overwhelmed with so many conflicting thoughts and emotions. I'm afraid to jinx the moment for fear he'll stop sharing so I smile wide and my eyes twinkle with unshed tears. I sit frozen and wait for him to continue, forgetting to breathe.

"I didn't say anything because I thought it hadn't been long enough and I worry the voices will come back," he adds.

We spend time talking and realize that one month after he started his thirteenth supplement, which happened to be magnesium, the voices stopped. This is so awesome and I immediately text my loved ones and tell them the astonishing news. Everyone is so excited and thankful we've passed this major hurdle. We know a true miracle is happening and we've recovered Daniel from severe mental illness. So many dear friends have loved ones struggling with the devastation of mental illness and I want people to know there's hope in the midst of turmoil.

While our family is finding peace and hope, there are so many families still caught in the turmoil of mental illness. I am so blessed to have an answer for my son and I believe the same answer can be applied to many others still struggling with mental illness. I'm saddened to hear that on October 29, 2014, a woman on Long Island was killed by her mentally ill son.[xlii] I can only imagine the trauma and threats this woman lived under while her son was free to walk the streets because she couldn't find care for him. There, but for the grace of God, go I. That this mom lived through this torment and died at the hands of her son grieves me more than I can express. The fact that a son can drag his mother out into the street after having decapitated her and throw himself in front of a train shows how little we have in the way of support for mentally ill families and their loved ones.

It's time for people to wake up to the trauma, torment and pain going on in homes all around the world. Families need help to deal with their mentally ill loved ones and the mentally ill need help to ease the torment going on in their minds. Most families suffer in silence because there's no one to talk to that understands what they're going through. The stigma is still so great in our country.

# Chapter Twenty:

# Keep My Son Heroic

———◆———

*So much of what is best in us is bound up in our love of family, that it remains the measure of our stability because it measures our sense of loyalty.*
*Haniel Long*

Christmas 2014 brings all our family together to celebrate. We hold our family close. We have all three children together with their spouses. Leonard and I know our lives are full and blessed.

We spend Christmas Eve at Tyler's in-laws, the Martin's, eating and playing a game called 'Heads Up' where you hold your iPad up against your forehead and your team sees the word and tries to get the person to guess it. We all laugh until our stomachs hurt. Daniel shines like a beacon and shows just how much he's retrieved his mind. During the game, I sit looking at Daniel with such pride that he didn't give up these last 19 years, and in fact is a perfect example of perseverance and determination. He's my hero. He didn't give up and take his life. Tyler sits next to me and has such a great time razing me for my non-stellar performance. It's wonderful to be laughing with all our loved ones; something that has been missing for decades is now returned to us.

The next day is Christmas and we head over in the morning to Tyler's home where our three granddaughters are excited to open presents. Tyler's father-in-law, Mac, comes to me to tell me he's surprised at the difference he can see in Daniel.

"Last year at Thanksgiving I was amazed at how well Daniel was doing, but this year I can see he has made a huge leap in recovery and I'm thrilled for all of you."

It makes me smile knowing that others who see Daniel infrequently can perceive his improvement. I look at Mac, and tell him, "It makes me so happy others can see what an improvement Daniel made this last year."

A few days later at church, I speak with a friend who came to our Christmas Eve dinner a few nights earlier and he also says, "Your son…it's amazing to see such a tremendous change in Daniel since I saw him the year before. What a miracle for Daniel's life." We're blessed to have our son back, and whole in mind.

Every month that passes Daniel improves steadily and we see more and more of our son from before the mental illness struck at age fourteen. I whisper my thanks to God for leading me and enlightening me to what I needed to do. Without His guidance and Him giving me strength, this never would've happened.

Fast forward one year and we are at Christmas morning 2015. It's such a dichotomy compared to 2009, and even better than 2014. What a change has been wrought in Daniel's health. It's hard to believe each year is an improvement from the year before. I remember worrying this wouldn't last and we would be thrust back into the chaos of mental illness and the stress that floods the lives of everyone who exist in it.

We meet at Tyler's home with Karis, and Daniel, along with their spouses and extended family. As we're watching the grandbabies open presents, Karis and Tyler are up to their old pranks and feeling playful on the sofa with their brother. I catch a rapid series of pictures of them. You can see their wheels turning and silent words passing between them. Of course, Daniel's catching the vibes too and is caught unaware that I'm taking pictures. I love these two photos of my children…to see Daniel laughing makes my soul shout with joy.

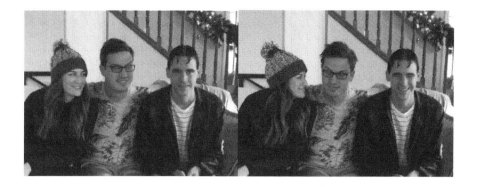

For me to say our son is well and the hallucinations, delusions, and voices are gone is a miracle. In my wildest dreams I never thought we'd see this moment happen. I thank God I was able to understand the process and implement the protocol for our son. Those with mentally ill loved ones know how hard it is to get compliance in anything from those suffering from mental illness. Our family is alive, Daniel is sane, and the voices that plagued him for so long are silent! Daniel has his mind back.

# Part Three

# CHAPTER TWENTY ONE:

# Methylation Pathway

———◆———

Part Three is for those who would like to know the steps I went through to recover my son from severe mental illness. This is my attempt to get it down on paper. I followed a specific protocol and implemented it carefully, as outlined by Dr. Yasko. I am indebted to Dr. Yasko for her brilliant and profound insight into the methylation pathway, and her tireless research. I don't mean to speak for Dr. Yasko, but from what I understand Dr. Yasko began working intensively with RNA/DNA in the 1980s, and in early 2000 turned her focus towards methylation, and neurological and autistic health issues. She's a pioneer in methylation and led the way for future doctors to also begin their journey learning about using this biochemical pathway, and implementing epigenetics (heritable gene expression-genes turned on or off), and nutrigenomics (the interaction of diet/nutrients and genes) in the healing process. Without Dr. Yasko, I'd have no framework for learning about this pathway or have any idea in how to go about tackling her system for myself and my son. She has a great network in place to help with questions and encouragement as you traverse this complicated pathway. All of her videos, books, manuals, protocols, diagrams, online support group, and analysis software are available on the web for free. I watched all of her videos repeatedly trying to absorb the words, learn the new language and try to make sense of it all. I sent in questions to the chat group, and they were quick to answer and give me sound advice. I read others questions and how Dr. Yasko's team answered their questions and just kept learning. Over time it really did begin to sink in.

Seven years later, I see the difference her research made in our lives. I hope those of you with loved ones who are suffering can make sense of the process and be strengthened and empowered enough to embark on this for yourselves. It's a journey worth taking and is life changing on so many levels. I encourage all of you to go to www.knowyourgenetics.com for the free learning material. Read, watch, read, ask questions…never stop. We're responsible for our own health and need to step up and start learning.

I am not a Ph.D., Doctor, Nurse, licensed, or certified. If I can learn this information and research, so can you. Immerse yourself in all of Dr. Yasko's amazing tools and jump in feet first, and don't look back. Take the time to educate yourself. This is a new beginning and a hopeful future from what you have known or lived before. What an exciting time to be alive and have this information at our fingertips. The research will, over time, lead us to a place where we can retrieve our loved ones from severe mental illness. It was a long journey, fraught with trial and error, steps forward and backward. The bottom line is that pursuing the methylation pathway biochemistry is key, and working on this for many years includes not giving up. I also realize as time goes on we'll learn more, and what we think we know now may change as methylation is understood at an even deeper level.

As I pursued care for Daniel over the last twenty years, I found the psychiatric medications prescribed by the doctors limited his mental illness but didn't make him completely well. The medications worked for a year or two and then the symptoms increased and the psychosis would break through again. When coupled with the nasty side effects of taking antipsychotic medications, you can see where following only the pharmaceutical avenue isn't an answer for many wanting a productive, coherent, and self-sustaining life. The coupling of the psychiatric medication and the nutrient levels needed by his body due to his genetics were a crucial link in returning Daniel to wellness. The Clozaril medication was instrumental in allowing me to work with him to bring about cellular repair in his body using nutrients.

I want to share what I did to recover my son to a point where he no longer hears voices after nineteen years. He's still on antipsychotic medications which helped to a point, but they didn't stop the voices, hallucinations, and delusions, and didn't get him to a grounded wellness. Clozaril was a game changer in that it turned off the addiction center in Daniel's brain allowing me to work with him to make the crucial steps in implementing the methylation protocol as laid out by Dr. Yasko. The prescription medications bring a degree of relief, but as you can see from Daniel's story, it's not full relief and it was always short lived. It's only with a combination of antipsychotic medications and nutrient supplementation specifically targeting his mutations lying on the methylation pathway that I was able to help get Daniel to a point of wellness where we no longer live in turmoil or fear. I never thought we'd achieve this goal. Remember when working with a mentally ill person it is a challenge. It's tough to get their buy in and compliance on treatment.

Many people who have the money and means run testing to find out the status of their nutrient and mineral levels, gut health, endocrine system, homocysteine, B12, Lithium, SAMe/SAH ratio, and heavy metal toxicity. It's important to address all of these aspects affecting your body and work at addressing all of the issues. Testing will help you pinpoint the issues and nutrient needs of your body. When we started on the methylation journey, Daniel was disabled and not working, so we didn't have the financial means to afford testing. Here are the steps I encourage you to follow:

1. Order Genetic Testing (can take up to 3 months to get results).

2. Pursue testing for legs 2 and 3 of the three legged-stool which is explained in Chapter 23.

3. While waiting for results, address glutamate/GABA balance in your diet and body. Check the glutamate containing foods and limit them if you're eating an excess of this type of food. Usually glutamate levels are higher in our bodies than GABA, which is a calming neurotransmitter.

4. Look at gut function (probiotics, digestive enzymes, pancreatic enzymes). Work with your doctor to heal your gut.

5. Check to see if heavy metal toxicity is an issue. Get tested and work with your doctor to detox your body.

6. Check to see if infectious agents are a problem. This includes Lyme. Get tested and work with your doctor to rid your body of pathogens.

7. Begin adding Step One nutrients from Dr. Yasko's supplement listing at Knowyourgenetics.com. These are important supplements for general wellbeing. For my son and myself, we ended up adding a lot of the Step One nutrients as we noticed big gains in our health just by adding these items. You'll also find many of the Step One nutrients are also the ones called out as beneficial for SNP function in Step Two because they're cofactors which help enzyme production at the SNP site.

8. Add one supplement at a time at a low dosage to see how you react.

9. Stay with one nutrient for four to six weeks and watch how you feel. Make note of how you react to the nutrient. If you react

poorly, reduce the dose, cut it in half, quarter, eighths, open the capsule and sprinkle some on food or in water, skip days, and be patient. You may find you just can't tolerate some nutrients. Stop them and try a different one from your list of options. You may find that at a later date you can try the nutrient again and you may be able to tolerate it as your methylation pathway is healing.

10.  Add the next supplement and follow the same steps in items 7 and 8 above.

11.  When your results arrive, download them and run them through any number of database options (listed later) which assess your raw data and provide reports.

12.  Address your genetic SNP mutations in a specific order of importance. As you begin addressing your mutations in Step Two, begin adding nutrients specific to SNP locations where you're at risk on the methylation pathway.

13.  This process takes time and patience. Remember, it took a long time to get where you are in your health and it'll take a long time to turn everything around.

# CHAPTER TWENTY TWO:

# What is Methylation

———◆———

Now let's dive in to how we recover our health. The first step is to learn about DNA and the methylation pathway.[xliii,xliv,xlv] Methylation is key in every cell in the body. Each cell in the body has to be able to accept and donate a methyl group ($CH_3$), which is a molecule made up of one carbon and three hydrogen atoms, with an available electron looking to pair up and cause a reaction. Methyl groups are highly reactive, and a reaction will occur, good or bad. It's this pairing up that turns on and turns off cells expression (i.e., turning off cancer cells, turning on apoptosis leading to cell death, etc.).

The knowledge we have to date shows us this process occurs on four separate but interconnected biochemical pathways, which Dr. Yasko describes as "wheels," that make up the methylation pathway and are intrinsic to every cell. The wheels don't move independently but instead drive each other. I like to envision them as gears in a watch where the teeth interconnect and push each other into motion. These pathways allow us to use nutrients and supplements to get around our SNP [(single nucleotide polymorphism)—pronounced 'snip'] mutations and get the pathway functioning at a better rate, thereby getting better enzyme function and turning on and off cell function as needed. Each SNP has a corresponding rsID code which is unique to its position on the DNA helix.

The four biochemical wheels are made up of the methionine, folate, BH4, and urea cycles. A fifth cycle, the Krebs cycle, intersects the urea cycle, where we see the ACAT SNP playing a role in methylation function. Each of these wheels are responsible for the function of well-defined nutritional genetic pathways. The first wheel—the methionine cycle—is key in the processing of B12, homocysteine, sulfur, ammonia, and is instrumental in the production of glutathione.[xlvi] The second wheel—the folate wheel—is key to the conversion of B vitamins and methyl group production. The methionine and folate wheels meet at a point where vitamin B12 is critical.[xlvii] Lithium helps drive the B12 into the cells so it's important to keep an eye on your Lithium levels.[xlviii]

The third wheel is the BH4 cycle. BH4 stands for tetrahydrobiopterin. This is a cofactor that is essential to makes you feel good and affects your brain neurotransmitter (serotonin, dopamine, epinephrine, and nor-epinephrine) levels. Your body needs BH4 to convert tryptophan and tyrosine into serotonin and dopamine.[xlix] Serotonin with enzyme catalysts forms melatonin.[l] If you have an overload of environmental toxins (such as lead, mercury, or aluminum), this can compromise the BH4 levels in your body.[li] Another factor which can affect your BH4 levels are bacterial infections. Knowing this, it's easy see how many aspects of our environment and our infectious load can affect our feel-good neurotransmitters. The gut is also called the second brain where 90% of your serotonin production occurs. Ensuring your gut is working optimally is key in regaining your health.[lii]

Lastly, the fourth wheel in the methylation cycle is the urea cycle. This wheel helps rid the body of ammonia.[liii] A lack of BH4 also affects this wheel and can cause neurological inflammation and damage.[liv] All four wheels are integral in the healthy functioning of the body and are part of the central pathway in every cell.

The methylation cycle is responsible for many functions in the human body and it's central to many critical reactions in every cell. Some of the reactions in which methylation is key include:

- Building and repairing DNA and RNA
- Energy production
- Metal detoxification
- Neurotransmitter balance
- Digestive issues
- Inflammation
- Myelination
- Cancer prevention
- Membrane fluidity

# CHAPTER TWENTY THREE:

# Other Factors Important to Health

———◆———

It's important to note there's more to your health than just your genetics. While it's key for us to recover our health, there are other issues you must address in order to make real inroads in healing your body. I like to envision regaining our health as a three-legged stool: 1) Genetic, 2) Environmental, and 3) Pathogenic. All three areas need to be addressed to recover your health. Many people trying to get well may find they've already addressed some of these areas with their doctor. Others will find this to be new information to think about and discuss with your doctor. Consider environmental factors affecting your body. Items such as your diet, histamine levels, stress, sleep quality and duration, heavy metal toxicity, and gut function all need to be addressed and improved. The third area of importance is your pathogenic load. Do you have bacterial, fungal, viral, and/or parasites which need to be treated? Working with your healthcare provider to look into all of these items will play a huge role in helping to restore you to a level where you can rejoin life and enjoy your family and friends. While our genetics put us at potential risk for the methylation cycle not running optimally, the other two areas addressed above are critical pieces of the equation and poor methylation will impact your ability to get legs 2 and 3 of the three-legged stool under control.

# CHAPTER TWENTY FOUR:

## Genetic Testing Sites

———◆———

Keeping in mind the four wheels of the methylation pathway, we're able to run a genetic test looking for mutations on this four-wheel biochemical pathway. The tests can be ordered by you through websites as indicated below. A doctor isn't needed to purchase the test kits. The test kit is delivered to your home and you retrieve the results from the testing site. There are options for SNP testing of your genetic DNA. I used three different testing sites over the last seven years in an attempt to find the cheapest way to get the SNP raw data and discover exactly what methylation SNPs are included in each of these packages.

The first site I used on our journey towards wellness was Dr. Yasko's site: www.holisticheal.com. For $495 (at the time of this writing) a test kit arrives at your home. The kit also contains reading material for you to begin learning about the methylation pathway while you wait for the results. The next step is to poke your finger and place three drops of blood on a piece of felt included in the kit, which you let air dry. You send your sample to the address included in the testing kit, and begin the wait for the sample to be analyzed. During the weeks while you wait for the results, immerse yourself in reading Dr. Yasko's research and watching her free videos. To date, there are thirty locations on key sites on the pathway that Dr. Yasko believes are critical for methylation and which lend themselves to testing and supplementation to bypass the mutations. I chose Dr. Yasko's test because while I was researching for an answer to our health crisis, I knew the complexity of the topic was immense and I was at a loss in how to go about implementing the program. I knew I needed the teaching materials in order to learn.

The second site I used was www.23andme.com. When I first ordered 23andme in 2012, I received all 30 of the methylation SNPs that doctor Yasko identifies as being at critical junctures in the pathway. In 2015, you now only receive 20 of the 30 SNP subset. 23andme keeps changing their vChip, which is a microarray chip used to detect SNPs. They are making it less and less attractive as an option for getting the methylation data we need.

At the time of writing this book, 23andme.com costs $199 and analyzes 600,000+ SNPs. This test kit also arrives at your home. It's a spit test that you mail back and then wait approximately nine weeks for the results. No learning materials are included and any information provided is not focused on methylation.

In 2015, I ordered from a third website, www.dna.ancestry.com, which costs $99 (at the time of this writing) and analyzes 700,000+ SNPs. It's a spit test that you mail back and wait nine weeks for the results. Unfortunately, you only receive 16 SNPs of the 30 SNPs subset which Dr. Yasko feels are needed. This number can change at any time if they adjust their vChip for analysis. No learning materials are included.

# CHAPTER TWENTY FIVE:

# Health is in your Hands

———————◆———————

When deciding to go down this road of using the methylation cycle to heal the body, you need to embrace the idea that your health is in your hands. You have choices you can make to help restore your health and you're responsible for making every effort to learn and implement what you learn. No one can hold your hand all the way through. It takes dedication on a personal level to tackle this process. You need to hunt down and find an excellent healthcare provider who isn't against learning cutting edge new ways to think about your health. Most physicians ignore and condemn nutrients as not helpful, ineffective, and not associated with healing, so finding a doctor that realizes food and nutrients are central to your wellness can be difficult. Don't give up. Walk away from those who won't help and keep hunting for a doctor that's willing to make the journey with you to wellness.

Doctors don't know what to do with this information as it's so new and they've not taken the time to learn about it yet. It can be very frustrating trying to find a care provider who'll walk this out with you. Yet as more and more people start expecting their doctors to be knowledgeable on this topic, we find that doctors and other caregivers are attending conferences to learn what to do and how to proceed in bringing health to their patients. Many people would say you can't do this, you'll make yourself worse. This wasn't my experience. Everyone has an opinion on how to proceed. You must do what you can in the situation you have - financially, physically and psychologically.

# CHAPTER TWENTY SIX:

## Layering in Nutrients for Step One

———◆———

While waiting for Daniel's genetic results, we began layering in supplements from Step-One of Dr. Yasko's protocol. As mentioned, the supplement list is available online at www.knowyourgenetics.com. This step layers in basic nutrients I assumed we were getting from our diet, but may not be.

A few months later, I was to find that our needs were greater than our diet provided due to our SNP genetic mutations. We proceeded very slowly and Daniel and I both watched for any inkling of an issue. We kept a log of the nutrient added and the date we started the supplement, making note of any and all symptoms we felt were notable. It was hard working with my son and his paranoid schizophrenia. Dealing with a person in a state of psychosis is very difficult. I measured every word I spoke, and encouraged him every step of the way. I didn't have the luxury of tackling all of the other issues that possibly were affecting Daniel. Trying to make a mentally ill person open to taking pills is a challenge unto itself. Getting Daniel to buy-in to going to numerous health appointments and submitting himself to expensive, time consuming visits wasn't going to happen. I decided we'll tackle his SNPs in the order outlined by Dr. Yasko (with a minor tweak in the order) and go very slowly watching for minor subtle reactions.

We began to add each supplement one at a time followed by a wait period of a month to six weeks or more between each nutrient to see how he felt. We kept an eye out in case he had a bad reaction to the new supplement. Dr. Yasko is a proponent of layering in small doses of supplements because some people can be very reactive to the smallest dose of a nutrient. We found this to be true when Daniel's general practitioner placed him on a prescription for Deplin 7.5mg, which is a therapeutic dose of L-5 methyl tetrahydrofolate (folate and a methyl donor). Don't mistake folic acid for folate. Folic acid is a man-made synthetic chemical.[lv] This simple B vitamin (folate), in a therapeutic dose, sent Daniel into a negative psychological tailspin. With this experience in hand, I too am now a big proponent of slowly layering in smaller doses and increasing this dose over time to hit a point where we're seeing favorable change.

# CHAPTER TWENTY SEVEN:

## Step Two After Results Arrive

———◆———

In the lingo of the mutation world, a mutation given by both mom and dad equals a double mutation, also called homozygous and shown as +/+. This situation is potentially more impactful and the enzyme at this location may be working at 20 to 30% of normal. If you receive a mutation from one parent, but a normal gene from the other this is called heterozygous and is shown at +/-. This situation may affect the enzyme at the location and it may be functioning at 60 to 70% of normal. A group of many heterozygous (single, +/-) SNPs may be as impactful as a homozygous (double, +/+) mutation.

When Daniel's test results arrived they showed that he had ten out of thirty (33%) of his methylation SNPs mutated. Daniel has double mutations (homozygous, +/+) on COMT V158M, COMT H62H, and VDR Taq (all tied to brain neurotransmitters). He also had single mutations (heterozygous, +/-) on MTHFR C677T, MTHFR A1298C, MTR A2756G, BHMT 01, BHMT 02, BHMT 04, and BHMT 08. Everybody has their own combination of mutations in the pathway and each person has a unique grouping of nutrients they need to address their individual SNP mutations. None of us are exactly the same and it is a very personalized approach to treating the methylation pathway in each individual.

When we found out Daniel's methylation pathway was compromised, we knew his system was in need of additional nutrient support to function properly in key areas. Dr. Yasko advises a person to start with ACAT, SHMT, and CBS in that order after laying down some of the Step One nutrients to help create a foundational level of wellness. Daniel's results showed he wasn't mutated on these three SNPs, so we knew to start with his double mutations downstream on the methylation pathway.

I decide to begin downstream in order to get the downstream mutations functioning optimally so they would be ready to accept the intermediates that would flow off of the four main wheels once we began addressing mutations located on the outer wheels and the crosscuts of those main wheels. My reasoning was if we didn't do the downstream SNPs first, the intermediates would become blocked behind the lower functioning downstream SNPs and cause a quicker build-up of intermediates (dopamine, serotonin, epinephrine, and nor-epinephrine) that couldn't process on through. This is the one area where I deviated from the Yasko Protocol. I laid out my theory with Daniel's doctor and he agreed that we tackle all of his downstream double mutations (COMT, VDR Taq) before turning our attention to the main pathway.

I realized the results meant nothing to Daniel, so we spent time together while I explained to him how the different SNPs affect the body's function. Information on each SNP and its function is available in Dr. Yasko's book Autism: Pathway to Recovery which is available on her website.

**CBS** (Homocysteine, Glutathione, Ammonia, Sulfur)

**ACAT** (Cholesterol, Lipids)

**SHMT** (DNA Building Blocks, Homocysteine)

**COMT** (Dopamine, Norepinephrine, Epinephrine)

**VDR** (Vitamin D, Dopamine, Blood Sugar Regulation)

**MAOA** (Serotonin)

**BHMT** (Methionine, Homocysteine)

**MTR** (Vitamin B12, Homocysteine)

**MTRR** (Vitamin B12, Homocysteine)

**MTHFR** (Folate, BH4)

**AHCY** (Homocysteine)

**SUOX** (Detoxify Sulfites)

**NOS** (Ammonia Detox of Urea Cycle)

After we finished reviewing Daniel's mutations, I knew I needed to proceed very carefully when implementing this protocol. Any wrong step and we all would pay a price of potential psychosis, which seems to always be looming over our heads. One wheel on the pathway can so easily affect another because they're interconnected. Daniel doesn't have any CBS, ACAT, or SHMT mutations, so we didn't have to deal with them. I began with his downstream mutations coming off of the four wheels and those were COMT, MAOA, and VDR Taq. The plan was to address the downstream double mutations (homozygous, +/+) first, and then address the downstream single mutations (heterozygous, +/-). We layered nutrients in one at a time. It took many, many months of watching to see how Daniel reacted and this determined how quickly we increased the very small doses. Finally, we were ready to move on after having added nutrients specific for the downstream SNPs.

I then turned my attention to the cross-cut SNP mutations (BHMT) on the methionine wheel by doing the same process of double homozygous mutations first, followed by single heterozygous mutations, at small doses metered in over time, at a slow pace while gradually increasing the dosage. Daniel and I sat at the formal dining room table and pulled out his methylation results and Dr. Yasko's diagram of the methylation pathway in order to look at each mutation and discuss if we'd addressed the specific mutations adequately or if we thought we needed to spend more time on a specific SNP by adding another supplement. It was a collaboration and we talked about all of our nutrient options which ultimately were approved by Daniel with his full support and compliance. This is a key step to the process because if he didn't buy into the decision, he wouldn't own the responsibility to follow through.

As the months moved forward, so did the improvements we saw in Daniel. It's rewarding to see the hard fought struggle of finding an answer to his devastating illness come to fruition and to help him come out of such a lost space mentally where there was no hope.

Once we addressed the downstream and cross cut mutations to an adequate level, determined by how Daniel felt, we decided to take the leap and turn on one of the four primary wheels where he had mutations. We held our breath and added the supplement known to activate the enzymatic process for MTHFR on the folate wheel. Since he's compound heterozygous for MTHFR (one mutation on C677T, and one mutation on A1298C), we knew turning on the folate wheel would force the movement of the other three wheels as they all drive each other. This is why we worked on the downstream and crosscut mutations first so these areas would be ready to receive the intermediaries coming off of the primary wheels when activated.

We were both uncertain and fearful that activating the primary wheel would cause the same issues we went through two years earlier when we first added Deplin to Daniel's medication line-up. With these worries in mind, we decided to use Fola Pro, an over the counter form of L-5 methyl tetrahydrofolate. We started with just one tablet, because we calculated that ten Fola Pro tablets equal one Deplin 7.5mg. We slowly worked up to six Fola Pro tablets and that was all he could tolerate due to his status as double mutated on COMT and double mutated on VDR Taq. People with these mutations are less tolerant of methyl donors. Fola Pro contains methyl donors so you need to be cautious when adding methyl folate. If you read the label on your nutrient bottle and see the term 'methyl' in the chemical compound, you'll know the product contains methyl donors.

We then continued to address his other mutations on the primary wheels and found that each step of the way, Daniel improved steadily and positively in all aspects of his health. We didn't have any backward steps, no crisis in health, and no psychosis. He began doing chores, his hygiene improved, and he was able to hold conversations, make eye contact, and talk freely. Once we finished adding supplements to address each specific SNP mutation, we decided to go back and add more basic nutrients from the Step One supplement listing of Dr. Yasko. We then also reinforced his double mutations (homozygous, +/+) by adding an additional nutrient to these SNP areas. We figured that strengthening the foundation of his nutrition would bring about even more profound wellness.

Finally, after two years, we found ourselves with Daniel hearing no voices, no longer living under a cloud of delusions, and seeing no hallucinations. It was a long, slow process but worth every minute. It's critical to stay with it, be patient, be consistent, don't give up, and know that it's a lengthy process back to health. You didn't get to this level of ill health overnight, and it takes time to heal the body and get cell function working optimally.

Stanford University published a study stating that every seven years we get a new body.[lvi] I like this idea because it reaffirms the process towards healing. Start now, and in seven to ten years you'll have a healthier you. Work on the three legged stool and methylation. If you do nothing to improve your health you will find a weakened body down the road.

We dealt with Daniel's SNPs and supplementation needs in order of mutation orientation on the methylation pathway wheels, and the nutrient list is below:

1. Hydroxy B-12 sublingual drop (Not a methyl donor)

2. Adenosyl B-12 sublingual tab (Energy production, not a methyl donor)

3. Multi-vitamin (All-in-One formulated for Methylation)

4. Vitamin B-150 (Complex of all B vitamins)

5. ACAT/BHMT Compounded

6. Probiotics

7. Wobenzyme-N (pancreatic enzymes)

8. Digestive Enzymes

9. GABA

10. Trimethylglycine (TMG) (Methyl donor)

11. S-Adenosylmethionine (SAMe) (Master methyl donor)

12. L-5 methyl tetrahydrofolate (Fola Pro)

13. Vitamin D3

14. Magnesium

15. Zinc Picolinate

16. Omega 3, 6, 9

17. Amino NR (Amino Acids)

When adding nutrients and supplements, always work with and defer to your doctor when choosing dosage and how to use the nutrients. I worked alongside Daniel's psychiatric team and his general practitioner letting them know each month what we were adding and the dosage. We planned ahead that if any of us saw any untoward reactions, we'd adjust the dosage to ensure success in bringing him back to great health. Thankfully, that didn't happen. On our journey we relied on each other to make sure Daniel continued to improve, and the outcome was amazing.

# CHAPTER TWENTY EIGHT:

## If I Could Dream...

————◆————

My heart's wish is that a well person from the family of the mentally ill would have the foresight to order a methylation pathway genetic test and begin the work of repairing the damage done by faulty performance of this biochemical pathway. After all, what if you too have mutations on your brain neurotransmitter SNPs (COMT, VDR Taq, and MAOA)? In an ideal world, mental health professionals would learn about methylation and the methylation pathway. It takes years to truly grasp the intricacies of this pathway and how powerfully it can be affected by nutrients.

I wish that people dealing with hallucinations, delusions and voices be given the option for placement on Clozaril very early in the process and not decades down the road when the mentally ill person has had numerous psychotic breaks affecting their brains, are homeless out on the streets, or have traumatized their family so much they're not welcome around their families anymore. Clozaril binds to serotonin and dopamine receptors which are important neurotransmitter, though they are often times a part of the problem if these neurotransmitters pile up too high in the body.[lvii] Not surprisingly, the neurotransmitters dopamine, serotonin, epinephrine and nor-epinephrine are also tied to the methylation pathway.[lviii]

Under a true health-care system, testing for this pathway would be covered by insurance. If the methylation pathway isn't working adequately, there will be a myriad of different health issues depending on the mutations specific to a person's body.[lix] It's in the insurance companies' best interests to support these tests, if for nothing else but for preventative medicine. The mentally ill are usually destitute and have lost their support structure because families are exhausted by efforts that don't come to fruition. The mentally ill don't have the resources for testing so they don't get the opportunity for the help that would be apparent if the testing was allowed and the cost was covered by insurance.

In addition, the nutrients and supplements required to bypass the mutations on the methylation pathway should also be covered by insurance. Why does insurance only cover the man-made, synthetic prescriptions that pharmaceutical companies make billions on, but not the natural substances of which pharmaceuticals drugs are often based? It's time to think outside the box. Insurance companies should be required to cover nutrients which are great healers of the methylation pathway and the body. I think about the money saved by the state now that Daniel is stable. The burden of the cost of the testing and all of his nutrients are born by us, not insurance. However, most families don't have the means to pay for this cost out of their own pockets. Daniel has not had a hospitalization since we started down this path. Think of the money saved if we could stabilize our mentally ill and ensure they and their loved ones were safe.

I wish you all the best on your journey. Don't ever give up. Remember, you are your own best advocate; no one cares about your health as much as you do. Seize the reigns and push ahead to your new future. Plan out your game strategy, chose a fantastic, open minded, willing medical team to walk with you. Don't be afraid to change out caregivers until you have the best group possible to help you regain your health. It's your money, your time, your health. Carpe diem and go forth with encouragement and fortitude!

# Appendix

# Resources

———◆———

## Websites:

www.Facebook.com/DrAmyYasko (Amy Yasko, Ph.D. Facebook Page)

www.CH3Nutrigenomics.com (Amy Yasko, Ph.D. discussion group)

www.DrAmyYasko.com (Amy Yasko, Ph.D. personal website)

www.scribd.com/DrAmyYasko (Amy Yasko, Ph.D. articles on Scribd)

www.DrAmyYasko.com/Resources (Amy Yasko, Ph.D. additional resources)

www.KnowYourGenetics.com (Amy Yasko, Ph.D. nutrigenomic analysis). Dr. Amy Yasko's website where the user supplies the data into the Neurological Research Institute platform to receive analysis of the SNPs and supplements to help bypass the effects of single and double mutations at the location of 30 different SNPs. You can also upload your 23andme raw data into this database and receive a 61-page report on your SNPs and associated nutrients that aid each individual SNP. Also, from this website you can access other numerous websites provided by Dr. Yasko. This is an awesome website to turn to for great research and resources. Dr. Yasko is gracious and allows access to her information free of charge.

www.MTHFRsupport.com Sterling Hill Erdei. Find a practitioner. Use her application to analyze your raw data results. Uses Livewello.com, accesses 23andme.com data to look at ninety-eight mutations (at the time of this writing) in the methylation pathway. This is an in depth look at other items besides methylation. The report shows your SNPs associated with mutations, known to date, that are potentially causing your body to have to work harder to perform activities associated with detox, IGA, IGE, IGG, allergy, clotting factors, gluten intolerance, mitochondrial function, other immune factors, sulfotransferase, thyroid, and tongue tie. This service charges a nominal fee. This information does not teach you about the methylation pathway, or how to implement a protocol to start supplementation. They do have doctors you can access for appointments to discuss health issues.

www.23andme.com   Less than $200 and analysis of almost 600,000+ SNPs.

www.dna.ancestry.com Less than $100 and analysis of 700,000+ SNPs.

www.geneticgenie.org Run 23andme raw data through this database and receive output that visually resembles Dr. Yasko's results. Donation requested for use of their database. They give you results on methylation and liver detoxification.

www.Livewello.com   Templates for analysis of SNPs associated with illness. Current cost is $20 for a lifetime membership. You can pay an additional monthly fee to access their ready-made templates on different health issues. They don't just concentrate on methylation.

www.Nutrahacker.com (Uses data results from 23andme.com)

www.walshinstitute.org (William Walsh, Ph.D. Nutrient Power – mental health issues)

www.mensahmedical.com (Albert Mensah, MD Advanced nutrient therapy) www.orthomolecular.org  The late Abram Hoffer, MD Orthomolecular approach to mental illness

www.orthomolecularhealth.com  Nutrition to help with mental illness.

www.truehope.com  Nutrient supplement product.

www.MTHFR.net  Dr. Ben Lynch. Find a doctor. Read his research.

www.functionalmedicinedoctors.com

www.md.com  (Choose Functional Medicine specialty)

www.myfunctionalmedicine.com

MTHFR Gene Mutation (Facebook group mediated by Dr. Carol Savage)

## Books:

Genetic Bypass by Amy Yasko, Ph.D., CTN, NHD, AMD, HHP, FAAIM (free on internet)

Autism: Pathways to Recovery by Amy Yasko, Ph.D., CTN, NHD, AMD, HHP, FAAIM (free on internet)

Feel Good Nutrigenomics by Amy Yasko, Ph.D., CTN, NHD, AMD, HHP, FAAIM (free on internet)

Feel Good Biochemistry by Amy Yasko, Ph.D., CTN, NHD, AMD, HHP, FAAIM (free on internet)

The Power of RNA by Amy Yasko, Ph.D., CTN, NHD, AMD, HHP, FAAIM

Mental and Elemental Nutrients by Carl Pfeiffer, MD

Molecules of Emotion - The Science behind Mind-Body Medicine by Candace B. Pert, Ph.D.

Nutrient Power by William Walsh, Ph.D. mental health issues.

# Health Issues Tied to Methylation

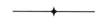

| | |
|---|---|
| Aging | Infertility |
| Allergies | Inflammatory conditions |
| Alzheimer's disease | Kidney failure |
| Anxiety | Lou Gehrig's |
| Arthritis | Low T Cells |
| Atherosclerosis | Lupus |
| Autism | Macular degeneration |
| Bipolar | Migraines |
| Bowel disorder | Miscarriages |
| Brain function | Mitochondrial disorders |
| Cancer | Neural tube defect |
| Cardiovascular disease | Nerve myelination |
| Crohn's disease | Neurological imbalance |
| Chronic fatigue syndrome | Neurotransmitter imbalance |
| Chronic viral infections | OCD |
| Diabetes | Pain Sensitivity |
| Digestive problems | Parkinson's disease |
| Dementia | Paranoia, panic attacks |
| Downs Syndrome | Psychiatric disorders |
| Fetal Development | Reduced NK cells |
| Gout | Rheumatoid arthritis |
| Heavy metal toxicity | Schizophrenia |
| Hormone deficiencies | Seizures |
| Immune Function | Skin conditions |
| | Thyroid disorders |

# Timeline of Daniels Illness

———◆———

Time line of medical episodes, medicines, supplements, response and outcome with Daniel that we dealt with during the twenty years of mental illness:

**Time Period; Episode; RX or Supplement; Response; Outcome**

**April 1995:** Daniel first shows signs of mental illness at the age of fourteen. Therapist: Woody. Medication: Prozac. Daniel isn't improving so he's sent to see a psychiatrist Dr. Donovan.

**Fall 1995:** Dr. Douglas Donovan threatens to remove Daniel from our home if harder drugs than marijuana and alcohol are found in his system. Medicine: Risperidone, Lithium, Effexor. Daniel not improving. Doctor authorizes use of marijuana and cigarettes. Diane not allowed to participate in appointments. Daniel isolated from family in this treatment style.

**Spring 1996:** Insurance changes at Leonard's work. Medicine: Risperidone, Lithium, Effexor. Daniel not improving. Becoming belligerent and more withdrawn. Daniel moved to a new psychiatrist.

**Spring 1996:** New psychiatrist Dr. Brian Pershall. Medication: Risperidone, Lithium, Effexor. Daniel improving slowly. Family invited to participate in Daniel's care to ensure honesty and accountability.

**1997:** Dr. Wilkinson. Allergy testing through National Biotechnology Laboratory. Allergies to dairy, bananas, plantain, chocolate, margarine. Supplements: Niacinamide, B12 shot/day, Selenium, Iron, DHEA, and slowly lowers his psychiatric medications. After Daniel cleans up his diet, he feels better. Dr. Wilkinson adds Inositol, Daniel goes off psychologically by evening and we can't get him back under control. Dr. Wilkinson pulls back from medical care for Daniel and advises us to work with his psychiatric team. Daniel is put back onto his regular dose of psychiatric medications.

**1999:** Medication change due to mental instability. Medication: Zyprexa started, Risperidone stopped. Responded well mentally on Zyprexa, but had a bad weight gain side effect (50 lb. increase). Only made it five months before stopping and going back to Risperidone.

**Fall 2000:** First psychiatric hospitalization. Seven-day stay. Medication: Risperidone, Lithium. Hallucinating, angry, paranoid, demons. Discharged as sick as when admitted.

**February 2002:** Second psychiatric hospitalization. Daniel walks in and asks to be admitted because he knows otherwise he'll die. Fourteen-day stay. Medication: Risperidone, Lithium. Drinking huge volumes of alcohol. Discharged as sick as when admitted.

**September 2003:** Daniel starts on True Hope supplement program. Multiple supplement blend, along with medication: Risperidone, Lithium. He does really well on the True Hope product when combined with his antipsychotics. Nutrient therapy improves his health.

**2004:** Daniel needs medication change as mental illness is worsening. Medication: Stopped Risperidone. Started Seroquel. Made too drowsy, can't stay awaken and will sleep 20+ hours. Stopped after a few months, goes back on Risperidone.

**2005:** Holter stress test for rapid heart rate of 190 bears/minute. Medication: Placed on Toprol, Zbeta and Atenolol trials.

Toprol and Zbeta are not tolerated due to anxiety, anger, and depression worsening. Atenolol works well and is prescribed.

**2009:** Daniel won't comply with directions from Grace Center, so they kick him out of their care. Medication: Risperidone, Lithium. Daniel says he's well and doesn't need psychiatric care. Ultimately, Daniel is transferred to New Hope under psychiatrist Dr. Patterson.

**August 27, 2009:** Third psychiatric hospitalization. Eighteen-day stay. During inpatient stay Dr. Namath prescribed Risperidone, Zyprexa Zydis, Lithium, and Valium. Upon discharge Daniel is prescribed medication: Risperidone, Lithium, Effexor XR, Zebeta, Iron, and Melatonin. Daniel says he's not sick and doesn't need care. Discharged as sick as when admitted.

**October 29, 2009** through November 16, 2009: Fourth psychiatric hospitalization. Fourteen-day stay. Medication: Invega Consta IM every 2 weeks, Zebeta, Antabuse, Melatonin. Daniel says he's not sick and doesn't need care. Discharged as sick as when admitted.

**December 2009:** Daniel is placed in the detox facility. Drinking alcohol while on Antabuse. Antabuse stopped. Extremely psychotic. Daniel is transferred to psychiatric hospital.

**December 2009:** Fifth psychiatric hospitalization. Twenty-three-day stay. Daniel is taken off Invega Consta injections. Medications upon release: Abilify, Zebeta, Melatonin, Folic Acid, Thiamine, multivitamin / multi-mineral, Cyanocobalamin B12. Extremely psychotic. Discharged as sick as when admitted. Awaiting an inpatient bed for a dual diagnosis program.

**January 2010:** Inpatient at Passages. This is a dual diagnosis program that runs for six weeks. Medication: Abilify, Melatonin, Zebeta, Folic Acid, Thiamine, multivitamin/ multi-mineral, Cyanocobalamin B12. One week after starting the program they call Diane to come get Daniel, because he won't participate. Kicked out of program for not participating.

**March 16, 2010:** Sixth psychiatric hospitalization. Two week stay. Medications on discharge: Abilify, Geodon, Cogentin, Zebeta, Melatonin. Extremely psychotic, placed in separate wing from other patients. Sent on to the State Mental Hospital.

**March 25, 2010:** Seventh psychiatric hospitalization. Daniel is admitted to State Mental Hospital. Daniel is kept inpatient from March to November. Medication on admission: Risperidone, Lithium, Effexor, Zebeta. Extremely psychotic. No change in psychosis.

**March 25, 2010:** Huge problem with the volumes and volumes of water or liquids that Daniel drinks. Medications: Risperidone, Lithium, Effexor, Zebeta. 24-hour presence of a worker to try to stop him from drinking fluids. No change in psychosis.

**April 3, 2010:** Medication change: Risperdal, Lithium, Zebeta. They stop Effexor as it's making him manic. No change in psychosis.

**April 8, 2010:** Daniel has thyrotoxicosis (hyperthyroid). Medication: Risperdal, Lithium, Zebeta. No change in medication. No change in psychosis.

**April 12, 2010:** Medication: Risperdal, Lithium. Daniel is removed from his beta blocker (Zebeta) in December as it can potentially make him depressed. No change in psychosis.

**April 27, 2010:** MRI came back negative on Daniel's brain. Medication: Risperdal, Lithium. No change in his care. No change in psychosis.

**May 12, 2010:** Medication change: Risperdal dose increased. The dose is divided into two doses throughout the day. No change in psychosis.

**May 8, 2010:** Medication change: Daniel states he was given Vistaril medication in a one-time dose that works for the rest of his life. Obviously this type of dosing isn't real. Not sure if it really happened. No change in psychosis.

**June 5, 2010:** Medicine change: to either Zyprexa or Haldol. Daniel isn't open to Zyprexa as it makes him gain weight. Starts Haldol. Daniel states he feels less anxiety. Psychosis still evident.

**July 5, 2010:** Medicine change: Starts antidepressant. Daniel states he feels better after first dose. No change in psychosis.

**August 14, 2010:** Medicine change: Only on Risperdal. Taken off of Haldol, Lithium and antidepressant. No change in psychosis.

**September 13, 2010:** Medicine change: Continues Risperdal, adds Haldol. Daniel is feeling less angry and has less violent thinking. Daniel stated he walked around feeling really angry prior to meds change, and feels the medicine is helping. No change in psychosis.

**October 9, 2010:** Medication change. Risperidone dosage decreased, Haldol same dose. No change in psychosis.

**October 23, 2010:** Medication change: Risperidone increased, Haldol same dose. No change in psychosis.

**November 2, 2010:** Released from State Mental Hospital. Medication: Risperidone dose unchanged. Haldol dose unchanged. Daniel released as sick as when he was admitted in March 2010. No change in psychosis.

**November 7, 2010:** Daniel was detained and taken to the Detox facility. Medication: Risperidone dose unchanged. Haldol dose unchanged. No budget for detox facility, so no bed. Discharged after a few days. No inpatient hospital bed available to treat psychotic behavior, so they can't transfer Daniel…we take him home. No change in psychosis.

**November 24, 2010:** Medication change: Remeron for depression and sleep aid. Daniel states he feels better on Remeron. He's sleeping a lot. No change in psychosis.

**November 30, 2010:** Daniel went to Emergency Room (ER). Threatened to kill Diane in front of a nurse. Security stood outside hospital door. No psychiatric bed available. Medication: Albuterol, prednisone. Acute bronchitis, cough, GERD. We took him home as no psychiatric bed available. No change in psychosis. His case manager is checking to see if Daniel is a candidate for Clozaril for treatment resistant schizophrenia. Criteria for acceptance is failure of two standard antipsychotics.

**Jan 2, 2011:** Medication change: Starts Clozaril. Continues Atenolol, Remeron, and Omeprazole. No drive for alcohol. Sober three days later.

**October 17, 2011:** MTHFR genetic test results arrive. Medication: Starts Fola Pro increasing to 10 tablets, switches over to Deplin. Two heterozygous mutations (compound heterozygous) for MTHFR. This genotype associated hyperhomocysteinemia and an increased risk for coronary artery disease and venous thrombosis. After 3 to 4 weeks, Daniel becomes quite sick and starts showing signs of anxiety, anger and isolation. We stop the Deplin.

**Spring 2012:** Ordered the Yasko 30 SNPs panel for the methylation pathway. Medication: Clozaril, Atenolol, Remeron, Omeprazole. Waiting for results. Reading literature and watching videos about methylation pathway. Daniel is willing and eager to start treating his methylation pathway if it will help him continue to improve.

**August 2012:** Methylation pathway mutations results are back. Medication: Clozaril, Atenolol, Remeron, Omeprazole. Daniel has 10 mutations out of the 30 possible. Holding off implementing protocol. Travel to Maine to learn more about methylation pathway.

**September 2012:** Diane and Leonard head to Maine to learn how to implement the methylation pathway protocol with Dr. Yasko. Medication: Clozaril, Atenolol, Remeron, Omeprazole. Ready to start the protocol for Daniel after 3-day conference.

**October 2012:** SNPs dealt with in order of location on the methylation pathway over the next two years. Medication: Clozaril, Atenolol, Remeron, Omeprazole.

**October 2012:** Supplement for SNP mutations COMT 158 & 62/VDR Taq, MTR 2756, BHMT 08. Supplements: Hydroxy B-12 drops for Basic Methylation. Three downstream SNPs and one crosscut SNP. Slowly increase B12 drops from once a day to twice a day.

**November 2012:** Step One. Supplement added: Multi-vitamin (Beyond Any Multiple – BAM; later switched to All-in-One).

**December 2012:** Step One. Supplement added: Vitamin B-150.

**January 2013:** Supplement for SNP mutations BHMT 01, 02, 04. Supplement added: ACAT/BHMT Compounded Capsule. Three crosscut SNPs.

**February 2013:** Step One. Supplement added: Probiotic. Good bacteria for gut health.

**April 2013:** Step One. Supplement added: Wobenzyme-n. Pancreatic enzymes for gut health.

**May 2013:** Step One. Supplement added: Digestive Enzymes. Enzymes to aid in food breakdown and assimilation.

**July 2013:** Step One. Supplement added: Gamma-aminobutyric acid (GABA). Anti-anxiety and calming.

**August 2013:** Supplement for SNP mutations MTHFR 1298, MTR2756, BHMT 08. Supplement added: Trimethylglycine (TMG). Two SNPs on primary wheels and one cross cut SNP.

**September 2013:** Supplement for SNP mutations COMT 158 & 62/VDR Taq, BHMT 08. Supplement added: S-Adenosyl methionine (SAMe). Three downstream SNPs and one crosscut SNP.

**November 2013:** MTHFR C677T. Supplement added: L-5 methyl tetrahydrofolate (Fola Pro) - start 1 tab/day increase to 6 tab/day over a 2-year period. One primary wheel SNP.

**December 2013:** VDR Taq/COMT 158 & 62. Supplement added: Vitamin D3. Three downstream SNPs.

**August 2014:** Step One. Supplement added: Magnesium. Key co-factor in the methylation pathway. Daniel no longer hears voices.

**September 2014:** Step One. Supplement added: Zinc. Key co-factor in the methylation pathway. Daniel continues to improve.

**January 2015:** Step One. Supplement added: Omega 3, 6, 9. Essential fatty acids. Daniel continues to improve.

**April 2015:** Supplement added: Amino acids to offset vegan diet and potential lack of proteins (Building block of proteins). Daniel continues to improve.

# Glossary

————◆————

Adenosylcobalamin – A natural form of B12 important in the energy cycle in the cell, along with aiding your muscles, DNA, and brain. The body must go through zero conversion steps in order to use it. Does not contain a methyl group.

Allele – One of two alternative forms of a gene that arises by mutations and are found at the same place on a chromosome, and are responsible for hereditary variation.

Cyanocobalamin – A synthetic form of B12 that contains a cyanide molecule. The body must go through 4 conversion steps in order to use it. The body then needs to rid itself of the cyanide molecule. Requires methyl groups to clear from your body.

DNA – Deoxyribonucleic acid. The molecular basis for heredity, formed in a double helix.

Epigenetics – The study of heritable changes that are not caused by changes in the DNA sequence.

Excitotoxin – Substances which excite neurons. Glutamate is a frequently found substance added into our food supply which is an excitotoxin.

Gene Mutation – A permanent change in the DNA sequence that makes up a gene, they have varying effects on health depending on where they occur.

Genetics – The study of how genes control characteristics, heredity and variation in organisms.

Genotype – The genetic makeup of the cell with reference to specific characteristics being evaluated.

Homocysteine – Non-protein amino acid. Implicated in heart attacks, strokes, and blood clots.

Hydroxycobalamin – A natural form of B12 important for detoxification of cyanide and scavenges nitric oxide (NO).

The body must go through 3 conversion steps in order to use it. Remedy for cyanide poisoning. Does not contain a methyl group.

Hyperhomocysteinemia – Abnormally high levels of homocysteine in the blood.

Methyl – Not tolerated by everyone. COMT and VDR Taq SNPs may cause sensitivity to methyl donors.

Methyl group – A molecule made up of one carbon and three hydrogen atoms to form CH3. Utilized in the body for transport of nutrients in fat soluble states and in epigenetic processes, turning genes on and off.

Methylation – The addition of a methyl group to a substrate such as an enzyme, or the substitution of an atom or group by a methyl group. Methylation takes place over a billion times a second in the body. Bio-chemicals are passing methyl groups from one to another.

Methylation cycle – Made up of four separate biochemical wheels (methionine, folate, BH4, Urea) which interact with each other within almost every cell in the body. Essential for a number of critical reactions in the body. Genetic weaknesses (mutations) in this cycle may increase the risk factor for a number of serious health conditions.

Neurotransmitters – Brain chemicals that carry a signal from one nerve cell to another via a synapse.

Nutrigenomics – The study of the effects of foods on our gene expression. Identifying and understanding molecular level interaction between nutrients and the genome.

RNA – Ribonucleic acid. Helps make proteins in the body. Controls cellular and chemical activities.

Schizophrenia – A chronic, severe, and disabling brain disorder that affects 1.1 percent of the U.S. population. Schizophrenics interpret reality abnormally, and affects how they think, feel and act.

SNP – Single Nucleotide Polymorphism (pronounced 'snip'). A DNA sequence variation occurring commonly within a population.

Toxin – Substance introduced in the human body that is unstable, and causes illness.

VDR Mutations – The vitamin D receptor (Taq and Fok). While these are associated with how your body uses vitamin D, the VDR Fok mutation is also associated with blood sugar regulation. Also, mutations at the VDR Taq site can affect dopamine levels.

# Acknowledgements

———◆———

This book is a work of passion and pain. To the people who stood by my side and encouraged me to not give up, I can't thank you enough. It took two years to write and rewrite. I want to give unending thanks to my extended family members who took the time to read the first draft and give me feedback. You were invaluable. We had many discussions about whether or not I should even write this book, and in the end we decided we needed to share our story in the hopes we could be of help to other families struggling with the same types of issues.

I want to thank my technical editor Elisabeth Potter for reading and editing my story. I know it was hard and there were times you had to put the book down and take a break. After the first read through you handed it back and said, "Don't give it back to me for a long time because I need to recover. I don't know how you and your family survived this." You braved the story and gave me great suggestions for making it better. Thank you for your dedication to the process.

Also, a great shout out to my dear friend and extended family member, Cynthia Rutherford, for the beautiful original water color artwork for the cover of my book. I gave you some snapshots of Daniel and you created a masterpiece. It's funny that Daniel has never allowed me to hang a picture of him in our home, yet he loves your watercolor and is proud to let me hang it in a place of honor.

# Endnotes

i    Eric Topol, MD, The Patient Will See You Now. Basic Books, 2015, p. 3.

ii    Ibid. pp. 23–24.

iii    Ibid. p. 22.

iv    Griffin, K. L., 2000, "Parental Break Time," The Milwaukee Journal Sentinel, February 28, p. 1G.

v    Amen, D. G., 2015, http://danielamenmd.amenclinics.com/why-spect

vi    Metzl, J. M., and K. T. MacLeish, 2015, "Mental Illness, Mass Shootings, and the Politics of American Firearms," *American Journal of Public Health*, 105(2), pp. 240–249.

vii    Papachristos, A. V., A. A. Braga, and D. M. Hureau, 2012, "Social networks and the risk of gunshot injury," *Journal of Urban Health*, 89(6), pp. 992–1003.

viii    Egan, T., 1998, "Where Rampages Begin: A special report; From Adolescent Angst to Shooting Up Schools," *New York Times*, June 14.

ix    Freeman, S., 2015, "Bipolar Suicides," *Bipolarlives.com*.

x    Booth, J. H., 2013, *A Voice out of Nowhere*, September 4.

xi    Denno, D. W., 2003, "Who is Andrea Yates? A Short Story About Insanity," *Duke Journal of Gender Law & Policy*, Summer 10(1).

xii    Shea, S., 2014, "Sheilla Shea Reveals Why She Stabbed Her 6-Year-Old Son To Death; True Crime Author Janice Holly Booth Weighs In: Shameless Plea For Attention Or Courageous Revelation?" *PRWeb*, Charlotte, North Carolina, July 3.

xiii    Yakas, B., 2014, "Mentally Ill Son Who Beheaded Mom Was Off His Meds," *Gothamist*, October 31.

xiv    James, D. J., and L. E. Glaze, 2006, *Mental Health Problems of Prison and Jail Inmates*, Office of Justice Programs, U.S. Department of Justice, Washington, D.C., December 14.

xv    Rotter, M., 2007, "Sexual Offenders with Mental Illness:
      Special Considerations for a Special Population," *Psychiatric
      Times*, September 1.

xvi   Dundas, B., M. Harris, and M. Narasimhan, 2007,
      "Psychogenic polydipsia review: etiology, differential, and
      treatment," *Current Psychiatry Reports*, 9(3), pp. 236–41.

xvii  Washington State Senate Committee Services, 2011,
      *Washington's State-Funded Mental Health Services, Staff Overview
      Briefing for the Senate Ways and Means Committee*, Olympia,
      Washington, January 31.

xviii Washington State Hospital Association, 2012, *Mental Health
      Funding*, January 12.

xix   Hiday, V. A., M. S. Swartz, J. W. Swanson, R. Borum, and H.
      R. Wagner, 1999, "Criminal Victimization of Persons with
      Severe Mental Illness," *Psychiatric Services*, 50(1), pp. 62–68.

xx    The National Center for Victims of Crime, 2012, *Child Sexual
      Abuse Statistics*, Washington, D.C.

xxi   Associated Press, 2013, "Kennedy's vision for mental health
      never realized," *USA Today*, October 20.

xxii  DARA Thailand, 2016, "Blood Alcohol Concentration
      (BAC)," *AlcoholRehab.com*.

xxiii National Institute of Health, 2014, *Epigenomics and Epigenetics
      Research*, National Cancer Institute, Epidemiology and
      Genomics Research Program, Bethesda, Maryland, April 17.

xxiv  Schizophrenia.com, 2010, *Schizophrenia Facts and Statistics*.

xxv   Kuebrich, B., 2012, "Card Sorting, Pot Smoking, Pleasure
      and One Gene COMT," *Neuroamer*, June 29.

xxvi  Caspi, A., T. E. Moffitt, M. Cannon, J. McClay, R. Murray, H.
      Harrington, A. Taylor, L. Arseneault, B. Williams, A.
      Braithwaite, R. Poulton, and I. W. Craig, 2005, "Moderation
      of the effect of adolescent-onset cannabis use on adult
      psychosis by a functional polymorphism in the catechol-O-
      methyltransferase gene: longitudinal evidence of a gene X
      environment interaction," *Biological Psychiatry*, 57, pp. 1,117–
      1,127.

xxvii Henquet, C., A. Rosa, P. Delespaul, S. Papiol, L. Fananas, J.
      van Os, and I. Myin-Germeys, 2009, "COMT ValMet

moderation of cannabis-induced psychosis: a momentary assessment study of 'switching on' hallucinations in the flow of daily life," *Acta Psychiatrica Scandinavica*, 119(2), pp. 156–160.

xxviii Seeman, P., 2009, "Glutamate and dopamine components in schizophrenia," *Journal of Psychiatry and Neuroscience*, 34(2), pp. 143–149.

xxix Wenthur, C. J., and C. W. Lindsley, 2013, "Classics in Chemical Neuroscience: Clozapine," *ACS Chemical Neuroscience*, 4(7), pp. 1,018–1,025.

xxx Meltzer, H. Y., 2010, "Role of Clozapine in Treatment-Resistant Schizophrenia," *Disease Management and Treatment Strategies*, pp. 114–128.

xxxi Meltzer, H. Y., 2012, "Clozapine: balancing safety with superior antipsychotic efficacy," *Clinical Schizophrenia & Related Psychoses*, 6(3), pp. 134–144.

xxxii Davis, C. D., and E. O. Uthus, 2004, "DNA methylation, cancer susceptibility, and nutrient interactions," *Experimental Biology and Medicine*, 229(10), pp. 988–995.

xxxiii Miller, A. L., 2008, "The Methylation Neurotransmitter and Antioxidant Connections between Folate and Depression," *Alternative Medicine Review*, 13(3), pp. 216–226.

xxxiv National Institutes of Health, 2016, "MTHFR, methylenetetrahydrofolate reductase (NAD(P)H)," *Genetics Home Reference*, U.S. Department of Health and Human Services, Bethesda, Maryland, May 17.

xxxv National Institutes of Health, 2009, *What is Schizophrenia?* NIH Publication No. 15-3517, National Institute of Mental Health, U.S. Department of Health and Human Services, Bethesda, Maryland.

xxxvi National Institutes of Health, 2016, *Epigenomics*, National Human Genome Research Institute, U.S. Department of Health and Human Services, Bethesda, Maryland, April 1.

xxxvii National Institutes of Health, 2016, "What are single nucleotide polymorphisms (SNPs)?", *Genetics Home Reference*, U.S. Department of Health and Human Services, Bethesda, Maryland, May 17.

xxxviii  National Institutes of Health, 2016, "What is the epigenome?" *Genetics Home Reference*, U.S. Department of Health and Human Services, Bethesda, Maryland, May 17.

xxxix  Sen, A., N. Heredia, M. C. Senut, S. Land, K. Hollocher, X Lu, M. O. Dereski, and D. M. Ruden, 2015, "Multigenerational epigenetic inheritance in humans: DNA methylation changes associated with maternal exposure to lead can be transmitted to the grandchildren," *Scientific Reports*, September 29.

xl  Kendall, S., 2012, "Methylation Deficiency: The Missing Component to Neurological and Immunological Recovery," *Presented at the American Academy of Anti-Ageing Medicine World Congress, Held in Las Vegas, Nevada*, December 12.

xli  Talty, C., and M. Dahlitz, "Pyrrole Disorder for Therapists," *The Neuropsychotherapist*, (3) pp. 58–66.

xlii  Fuller, N., K. Deutsch, 2014, "Nassau cops: Farmingdale man with history of mental illness kills mother, then self," *Newsday*, October 29.

xliii  Medical News Today, 2015, "Schizophrenia-associated genetic variants affect gene regulation in the developing brain," December 1.

xliv  Phillips, T., 2008, "The role of methylation in gene expression," *Nature Education*, 1(1) p. 116.

xlv  Jin, B., Y. Li, and K. D. Robertson, 2011, "DNA Methylation Superior or Subordinate in the Epigenetic Hierarchy?", *Genes & Cancer*, 2(6), pp. 607–617.

xlvi  Belalcázar, A. D., J. G. Ball, L. M. Frost, M. A. Valentovic, and J. Wilkinson, 2013, "Transsulfuration Is a Significant Source of Sulfur for Glutathione Production in Human Mammary Epithelial Cells," *ISRN Biochem*, March 6.

xlvii  Fowler, B., 1998, "Genetic defects of folate and cobalamin metabolism," European Journal of Pediatrics, 157 Suppl. 2, pp. S60–S66.

xlviii  Schrauzer, G. N., K. P. Shrestha, and M. F. Flores-Arce, 1992, "Lithium in scalp hair of adults, students, and violent criminals. Effects of supplementation and evidence for interactions of lithium with vitamin B12 and with other trace elements," *Biological Trace Element Research*, 34(2), pp. 161–176.

xlix Wishart D. S., C. Knox, A. C. Guo, S. Shrivastava, M. Hassanali, P. Stothard, Z. Chang, and J. Woolsey, 2016, "Sapropterin," *DrugBank*, May 23.

l R. Delorme, J. Callebert, H. Goubran-Botros, F. Amsellem, .X Drouot, C. Boudebesse, K. Le Dudal, N. Ngo-Nguyen, H. Laouamri, C. Gillberg, M. Leboyer, T. Bourgeron, and J-M. Launay, 2014, "The serotonin-N-acetylserotonin–melatonin pathway as a biomarker for autism spectrum disorders," *Translational Psychiatry*, 4(11), p. e479.

li Robert, J., 2016, "Methyl Cycle Nutrigenomics," *heartfixer.com*, May.

lii Hadhazy, A., 2010, "Think Twice: How the Gut's 'Second Brain' Influences Mood and Well-Being," *Scientific American*, February 12.

liii Siegel, G. J., B. W. Agranoff, R. W. Albers, S. K. Fisher, and M. D. Uhler, editors, 1998, *Basic Neurochemistry: Molecular, Cellular and Medical Aspects, Sixth Edition*, J. B. Lippincott & Co., Philadelphia, Pennsylvania, November 1.

liv McNeill, E., and K. M. Channon, 2012, "The role of tetrahydrobiopterin in inflammation and cardiovascular disease," Thrombosis and Haemostasis, 108(5), pp. 832–839.

lv Schaefer, A., and P. Pletcher, 2015, "Folate vs Folic Acid," *Healthline*, July 21.

lvi Stanford Medicine, Institute for Stem Cell Biology and Regenerative Medicine, Stanford, California.

lvii Glatt, C. E., A. M. Snowman, D. R. Sibley, and S. H. Snyder, "Clozapine: selective labeling of sites resembling 5HT6 serotonin receptors may reflect psychoactive profile," *Molecular Medicine*, 1(4), pp. 398–406.

lviii Oh, J. E., N. Chambwe, S. Klein, J. Gal, S. Andrews, G. Gleason, R. Shaknovich, A. Melnick, F. Campagne, and M. Toth, 2013, "Differential gene body methylation and reduced expression of cell adhesion and neurotransmitter receptor genes in adverse maternal environment," *Translational Psychiatry*, January 22.

lix   Liu, L., T. van Groen, I. Kadish, Y. Li, D. Wang, S. R. James, A. R. Karpf, and T. O. Tollefsbol, 2011, "Insufficient DNA methylation affects healthy aging and promotes age-related health problems," *Clinical Epigenetics*, 2(2), pp. 349–360.

50221057R00175

Made in the USA
San Bernardino, CA
16 June 2017